Coping with Alzheimer's:

A Caregiver's Emotional Survival Guide

Rose Oliver, Ph.D.
Frances A. Bock, Ph.D.

Melvin Powers
Wilshire Book Company
12015 Sherman Road
North Hollywood, California 91605

To Juan
*Who forgot a great deal, but never forgot
the meaning of love.*
R.O.

To Hal
*Whose unique support and devotion
will always be gratefully remembered.*
F.A.B.

First Edition

1 2 3 4 5 6 7 8 9 10

Library of Congress Cataloging-in-Publication Data
Oliver, Rose.
Coping with Alzheimer's.

Includes bibliographies and index.
1. Alzheimer's disease—Popular works.
2. Alzheimer's disease—Family relationships.
3. Adjustment (Psychology) 4. Rational-emotive
pyschotherapy. I. Bock, Frances A. II. Title.
[DNLM: 1. Adaptation, Psychological—popular works.
2. Alzheimer's Disease—psychology—popular works.
3. Home Nursing—psychology—popular works. WM 220
048c]
RC523.045   1987   618.97'683   87-20213
ISBN 0-396-08933-X

Contents

Acknowledgments

We wish to acknowledge our debt to Dr. Albert Ellis, Director of the Institute for Rational Emotive Therapy, 45 East 65th Street, New York City. Dr. Ellis, psychologist, theoretician, and teacher, taught us that human beings, uniquely endowed with the ability to reason, can use that reason to solve emotional problems.

Rose Oliver, Ph.D.
Frances A. Bock, Ph.D.

Preface

Rational Emotive Therapy (RET) is the model that provides the underpinnings for this book. RET is a theory of human emotions, a system of psychotherapy, and a philosophy of life. It was originated over twenty-five years ago by the psychologist Albert Ellis, and today it is the leading theory in the ever-expanding field of cognitive-behavioral psychology.

As a theory of human emotions, RET, to a considerable extent, demystifies the realm of feelings. It explains the relationship between thoughts, feelings and behaviors.

As a system of psychotherapy, RET specifies *how* we can change our feelings by changing our perception of events, thus facilitating emotional and behavioral growth.

As a philosophy of life, RET holds forth the possibility that human beings, though fallible and imperfect, can live satisfying lives in a world that is imperfect and often painful.

How does this relate to you, the caregiver of an Alzheimer patient?

RET can show you how to identify and change your own dysfunctional emotional and behavioral responses. It can help you to learn to live with the reality of your loved one's Alzheimer's Disease (AD). RET can help you to maximize the quality of care for your afflicted relative while minimizing the emotional cost to yourself.

In the chapters that follow, we will refer to the principles and practices of RET under several different names: cognitive change, cognitive restructuring, changing dysfunctional self-talk, changing one's inner dialogue. The model is the same: You largely generate your own feelings. And you can change them. We will show you how.

Introduction: For You, the Caregiver

This book is for you, the caregiver. You may be young, you may be in the prime of life, you may be getting on in years. You may be raising young children, you may be struggling with the pain of separation from grown-up children, you may be excited with the prospect of the freedom from the cares of child-rearing that their departure will give you. You may be facing the problems and pleasures of the transition from young adulthood to middle age, you may have left middle age behind and are now coping with your own aging. You may be well, you may be ailing. You may be working, you may be a full-time homemaker. You may have plenty of time and money, both time and money may be in short supply.

You may be a husband, a wife, a daughter, maybe a son or a daughter-in-law, or possibly a niece or a granddaughter. What you have in common is a close relative with Alzheimer's disease, or a related disorder. This relative is dependent upon you for his care. You are one of millions of Americans. As more and more people live longer and longer, there will be more of you.

Each situation is unique. You bring to your own situation your lifetime experiences, your present reality, your hopes, dreams, wishes, needs, loves, and hates, as well as your patient's reality, his deteriorating mental and physical condition.

We will say little about caring for the victim of the disease. There are a number of excellent books on the subject. Some are listed in the References section at the end of this book. We will talk about the victim only insofar as his symptoms, behaviors, and needs impinge upon your life and create situations that you must address.

This book is for you. It will help you to deal with your thoughts, your feelings, your actions. It will show you how to do the best you can for yourself, in a situation that is at best, sad, at worst, tragic.

PART I

You Feel the Way You Think

CHAPTER **1**

The Logic of Feelings

Between the first signs of death of the mind to the final death of the body, some three to fifteen years later, there is a long road of agony for the family of the victim of Alzheimer's disease, particularly for the primary caregiver.

You, the caregiver, now find yourself thrust into a situation that threatens to overwhelm you with a welter of conflicting emotions and to undermine your ability to cope. At least, that is how it feels to you at times.

It seems that nothing in your life has come close to preparing you for what you experience daily as you struggle to do the best you can for your deteriorating family member. In this book we hope to show you how you *can* cope, despite the stress, the frustration, and the very real difficulties of your situation. We hope to show you how you can learn to do the best for yourself while doing your best for your afflicted relative.

The first step is understanding how your emotions

come about. Emotions—feelings—have their own logic, following their own set of rules. That may sound strange because you have probably grown accustomed to separating feelings from logic, as if they were unrelated, or even opposites. But in reality, you have been using these rules all the time, without awareness, to control and change your feelings. We all do.

Here is an example, based on everyday events, to show you how the logic of emotions works:

Joan is feeding her ten-month-old daughter when the phone rings. She speaks to the caller briefly, then returns to the high chair to find that the baby has made a mess by trying to feed herself. Joan smiles, thinking to herself, "How adorable." She feels pleased and happy.

Now, how did that happy feeling come about? Was it because of the baby's actions? Most people would say "Sure," and, in part, that is true. But it is not the whole story. The most important part has been left out.

Suppose Joan returns from the phone call preoccupied because her husband asked her to run an important errand right after lunch. Seeing the baby's mess, she thinks "Oh, no! I have no time for this now! Just when I have so much to do." Instead of feeling pleased, she feels tense, annoyed, frustrated. Yet the baby's actions are the same.

The missing element—the most important key to understanding Joan's feelings—is how she viewed the baby's actions and what she told herself about them. When she viewed the baby's actions as cute, she felt pleased, but when she viewed them as unwelcome or inconvenient, she felt highly displeased.

Her feelings, then, came about not primarily because of what occurred, but because of how she viewed those events—her own inner dialogue or the statements she made to herself.

Your feelings arise the same way—good ones and bad, sad, happy, or angry feelings, feelings of comfort or feelings of fear—all can be traced not solely to the events that triggered or activated your self-talk, but also to the inner dialogue itself.

Usually this inner dialogue makes pretty good sense—it sticks to reality, it rarely exaggerates or goes to extremes, and it would probably get general agreement or consensus from most reasonable people. Who would argue with Joan, for example, when she told herself that her baby's attempts at self-feeding were ill-timed and unwelcome and that she would have preferred something different? Even though Joan's feelings were negative ones of displeasure or annoyance, they were appropriate under the circumstance.

But sometimes our inner dialogues don't make good sense. They contain commands or demands rather than preferences, statements that don't square with reality and can't be supported by any evidence, statements that are extremes and exaggerations. When this happens, our feelings are inappropriate and so, usually, is our behavior.

Imagine Joan talking to herself about the same events like this: "Oh, my God, how could she do this to me? I can't stand this mess. This shouldn't have happened to me. Now I'll never get to the errand Alan wanted me to do and the whole day is completely ruined."

Instead of appropriate displeasure, now Joan feels inappropriately angry and upset. Her self-talk is dysfunctional, and she overreacts emotionally. The stage is set for a complicated cycle of inappropriate emotions, ineffective behavior, more dysfunctional thinking leading to additional emotional turmoil, and so on.

Let's follow Joan a bit further: She feels upset and angry, so she screams at the baby, who starts crying, thus adding another stressful element. Joan is so rattled by now that she turns over the milk container standing at her elbow. When she sees the mess that she added to what the baby had done, she thinks, "What a total idiot I am, not to mention an awful mother. Look how horribly I upset my child. I should be able to manage things better." Just then her neighbor comes in, realizes it isn't a good time to visit and excuses herself. Joan thinks, "What must she think of me? How could I let her see the house like this?" Later that afternoon, while out doing her errands, she remembers the phone call from her husband that started everything. She tells herself that he has no right to make so many demands of her and that he must, absolutely must, never bother her that way again. He comes home from work that evening unprepared for the angry diatribe Joan unleashes on him as soon as he opens the door. Not surprisingly, they say little to each other during dinner, and he soon finds some paperwork with which to busy himself until quite late. Joan goes to bed early—by herself—feeling quite lonely and unloved. She has run the gamut of emotional overreactions, from anger to shame, guilt and worthlessness, to lonely misery and despair. No wonder she's exhausted!

Did Joan have any other choice? Could she have chosen to feel and act differently, to stop upsetting herself needlessly, and to change her emotions? Could she have altered this unfortunate scenario? We believe the answer is Yes. We believe she could have listened to her self-talk and sifted the sense from the nonsense. By challenging her dysfunctional thoughts and replacing them with more reasonable self-statements, she could have helped herself to feel and behave more calmly and appropriately. She could have short-circuited her distress at any point in the sequence if she had known how to do so.

There are some important differences, as well as similarities, between Joan's situation and yours. She could have felt pleased by viewing events differently; this is not in the cards for you. It would be neither appropriate nor reasonable for you to feel pleased about your own or your family member's situation. But anger, despair, shame, and guilt didn't help Joan, and they won't help you. She didn't have to continue feeling that way, and neither do you. She could have applied the rules and the logic of feelings—and so can you.

This is the model of emotional change and choice that we will present in this book. It is based upon three simple assumptions:

(1) *You* generate your own feelings. They do not come out of the blue, nor are they predetermined by external events or other people.

(2) You feel pretty much the way you think.

(3) While it is human to get upset at times, you do not have to go on feeling overly anxious, angry, or depressed. You can change your emotions if you choose. This does not mean that your feelings are "right" or "wrong," only that they can be helpful or unproductive and that they can be changed.

We all carry on a more or less continuous dialogue with ourselves. We describe, analyze, judge, and evaluate people, things, and events. We say, "That's pretty," "That's ugly," "That's good," "That's awful," "I hate that," "That's easy," "That's too hard." Just monitor yourself for a day or so. You can make your own list of what you tell yourself throughout the day.

Some of the statements that you make to yourself are neutral in content; some have emotional consequences. Some self statements are adaptive; others are maladaptive. Adaptive thoughts are generally accurate and objective and generate feelings that motivate behaviors that are in your best interest. Maladaptive thoughts may be gross exaggerations, irrelevancies or overgeneralizations that generate emotions that impair your ability to function most effectively.

You will notice that when you say "That's great" or "That's beautiful," you get a little surge of good feeling. If you say "I can't stand that another minute," you are likely to feel upset. If you tell yourself that others should not behave in ways that you find unpleasant or obnoxious, you will probably feel angry. If you tell yourself that life is awful and horrible, you are likely to feel anxious and depressed. If, on the other hand, you remind yourself that there is no law on heaven or earth guaranteeing you a "happily ever after," you will probably weather the tough times with greater equanimity.

In the chapters that follow, you will read about situations typical in the lives of caregivers of Alzheimer patients. These situations will undoubtedly be familiar to you. So will the feelings of depression, anger, guilt, shame and loneliness. But something new has been added: We will help you tune in to your inner dialogue, to spot the unhelpful messages you give yourself, and to change them. We will help you learn the logic of feelings and make it work . . . for *you*, the caregiver.

CHAPTER **2**

Denial: A Limited Coping Strategy

How long has it taken you to admit to yourself that something serious has gone wrong with your spouse, your parent, your grandparent? How long did you delay getting a diagnosis, pretending that he was simply overworked, overtired, or just getting old? Or, if you were given a diagnosis of Alzheimer's or a similarly debilitating disease, how long did you try believing that your relative's problems weren't getting worse, didn't really impact on your life, and could be easily ignored? How many unmanageable situations have you gotten yourself into on the slow path toward acceptance of reality?

It's human to deny what we find unpleasant or frightening. We all tend to do it, and up to a point, it is adaptive to do so. Denial helps us not to worry about possibilities that may not materialize. It helps us to absorb the slowly changing behavior patterns of a person who had been familiar to us, but who now, at times, seems strange, erratic, unpredictable. It helps us slowly to integrate observations that we are not yet prepared to name, to categorize, to explain. But when new adaptations based on realistic evaluation of the situation are required, denial is maladaptive. It prevents us from seeking the facts or facing their implication. Like Ed, for example.

Ed was taken aback the first time a check bounced. He discussed it with Evelyn, and she said it must be a mistake. She would take it up with the bank.

Ed had noticed that Evelyn was getting a little absentminded lately. Once he found his socks in the refrigerator, and another time Evelyn looked at her sister Sylvia, who had come for dinner, and said, "Who are you?" But the next minute she offered her sister a drink, and everything seemed O.K. Ed laughed to himself and said, "Evelyn is losing her marbles." He didn't really mean it. It was just an expression.

But when the bank called Ed at work and told him that all his checks were bouncing, he realized something had to be wrong. He had always given Evelyn his paycheck to deposit. She watched the family budget, apportioned the cash, and paid the bills. She had always been very careful, very methodical, and generally managed to save something for a rainy day. Why were the checks bouncing? Ed looked in the checkbook. No deposits for four weeks.

Evelyn insisted that the bank was doing something to mess them up. Ed called the bank. There had been no deposits for four weeks. Where were the checks? Then Evelyn changed her story. They were stolen.

Ed searched the apartment. The checks were all in a brown bag in a kitchen closet.

Ed was furious. He vented his rage on Evelyn. What kind of game was she playing? Didn't she realize that she was getting them into all kinds of trouble? What could he tell the bank? How could he face all the people who received his bad checks? What could he tell his boss about his paychecks not being deposited? What else had Evelyn done that would come back to haunt them? He told Evelyn that he could no longer trust her, that she was totally irresponsible.

Evelyn was crushed. She insisted that she knew nothing about the checks in the brown paper bag. She couldn't remember anything about them. She started to cry and said that she was leaving, she couldn't stay another minute.

Slowly, Ed began to realize that Evelyn really didn't know anything about the checks. Slowly, he realized that the Evelyn who put the checks in the brown paper bag was not the Evelyn he had known for thirty years. He was bewildered.

Was she really "losing her marbles?"

He discussed the problem with Evelyn's sister. She said it must be her "changes." Women sometimes do funny things when they are going through their "changes."

Sometimes, well-meaning friends and relatives do their best to reinforce your denial or to thwart your efforts to face the facts. They can't believe that Jim, with whom they just had dinner, could possibly have lost his way when driving home. He surely must have business worries. Or that Selma looked at a raw chicken and didn't know what to do with it. After all, she was a pretty good cook! Surely you must be exaggerating. Everyone is forgetful sometimes.

What confuses people is that dementia, the mental deterioration characteristic of Alzheimer's disease, is neither unitary nor stable. It affects some functions sometimes and not others; it seems to fluctuate. If Jim lost his way home one night, he will not necessarily lose his way home every night. Evelyn may not recognize her sister one moment and act quite competently the next. Dementia may, in its early stages, affect one ability such as recognition of faces, or recall of names, and not others. This compounds the difficulty for you and your friends. At times, the Alzheimer's patient seems intact, and you doubt your own judgment. Other people often add to your doubts by assuring you that they see nothing wrong. So you continue denying and don't seek help when it would be appropriate to do so.

On the other hand, friends or relatives sometimes do try to point out to you that something is really amiss and suggest that you look into it. Either you don't hear them, or you don't want to hear them. You only hear what you are ready to accept. Acceptance is not easy. It necessitates many adjustments that you may not be prepared to make. Until, like Beth Williams, reality forces you to face the facts.

Beth's father, a widower and retired engineer, had until recently led an active and independent lifestyle. He had his own friends, his own interests, and he was a source of strength and wisdom to his recently divorced only daughter. When Mr. Williams grew forgetful, inactive, and reclusive, Beth denied there was anything wrong. That helped her keep her fears at a distance. She felt better . . . for a while. But her father's behavior continued to deteriorate. The demands of keeping up his own apartment grew more difficult for him. Dirty clothing began to pile up in a heap in the bedroom, leftover food was strewn about the kitchen, and the once well-stocked refrigerator was sometimes empty. Friends suggested to Beth that she arrange for housekeeping assistance, but she insisted that that would be "babying" him. It was just a phase. He'll get over it.

One night, she received a call from the police. Mr. Williams had been found wandering about two miles from home, dazed and confused. The police brought him home to an apartment in disarray. The time had come for Beth to face reality. Her father could no longer be left alone to fend for himself.

Clearly, Beth's denial was contrary to her father's best interests. But what about her own? How did it help her to perpetuate the illusion that her father was not, in fact, dementing?

Let's open an imaginary window to Beth's mind and listen to her thoughts about her father and herself:

"I've always looked to Dad for guidance and strength. He's always been there for me whenever I've had a problem, especially since the divorce. He's always been so wise and so helpful. I know that people sometimes get senile, but not Dad! Not my father! I don't know how I can handle things without him. The thought of having to take care of him as well as myself—well, it just terrifies me."

Did Beth really alleviate her own distress by refusing to accept the accumulating evidence of her father's deterioration? It seemed so at first. While Mr. Williams was still able to keep his own apartment, Beth's denial helped her not to "awfulize" about what might happen to him, and to her.

As his deficits increased, however, Beth's denial grew less and less adaptive. It was then that her dysfunctional inner dialogue became a real problem, generating her excessive fears. She responded in the only way she knew—more denial. She tried to quell her fears by pushing them away. In order to do that, she denied what had become obvious to others. Beth found it hard to give up the strategy that had seemed to work so well for so long, especially since no other was readily available—or so she thought.

At this point, Beth was simply sticking Band-aids on her distress, which continued to fester underneath. The signs of her distress included fatigue, irritability and impatience leading to friction with her friends, and a worsening of her hypertension, necessitating higher doses of medication. These hidden costs of denial weren't as apparent to Beth as was the temporary relief she got by avoiding rather than facing her fears. She was denying not only the facts about her father, but her own feelings as well. Her denial hurt rather than helped her to accept her emotions and come to terms with them.

To *truly* alleviate her distress, Beth had to learn to examine her self-talk and change much of it—especially the parts about "needing" her father to remain the strong parent and the absolute "impossibility" of her being able to manage her own life, along with his care.

We will return to the issue of dysfunctional self-talk in later chapters and show you better long-term coping strategies than denial. We will show you how to give up your maladaptive inner dialogue and to substitute more appropriate self-enhancing and realistic perceptions of your situation. The important point for you to remember here is that denial, while appearing to have short-term benefits, doesn't help you in the long run.

For example, Amanda Fischer's reluctance to accept the reality of her husband's illness led her to make a pretty costly mistake. Amanda and Bill had been married for thirty-five years when Bill was diagnosed as having Alzheimer's disease. The familiar early signs of memory loss, confusion, inability to keep up with

hobbies and friends we.
was made in the usual
sibilities.

Bill occupied himself put.
suburban home, while Aman.
writing. For a while, there
though she had been told that
was progressively deteriorative,
that he had stabilized. She wa ... ... to
believe that this was true, so she c. .adictory
evidence. For instance, although i. .vas generally
quiet and manageable at home, he became overwhelmed and upset over the slightest change in routine. A short trip into the city to see a play turned
into a fiasco when Bill got up during the first act,
loudly announced he had no intention of sitting through
such a poor performance, and continued to complain
in the lobby until their hired car returned to take
them home.

Nevertheless, Amanda rented an expensive beach-
front cottage for summer weekends. She told herself
that Bill had always loved the ocean, and even though
he could no longer sail, it would be nice for him to
walk along the beach. She gave little importance to
the packing, the traveling, and the change to unfamiliar surroundings that her plans would entail. She
didn't mind taking all the responsibility herself. She
allowed her thoughts to dwell on the lovely weekends
they would have, the friends who would join them,
the cookouts, maybe a clambake.

The first weekend, after she unloaded the station
wagon, Bill had his first "catastrophic" reaction. He
accused her of being a spy, of taking him out of the
country, of hiding his camera . . .

Amanda was forced to face the facts. Bill's illness

transient nor stabilized. It was deterio-
life would no longer be the same.

ter the first nightmarish weekend, Amanda tried
to cancel the rental. Too late. Too bad. She had to forfeit a sum of money she could ill afford to lose. Like Beth, Amanda had stayed with a limited strategy for too long. It was an expensive mistake.

Amanda learned an important lesson, however. She learned to stop denying the evidence of Bill's decline and to accept her own feelings as well. In the aftermath of her collapsed summer plans, she felt disappointed, apprehensive, and angry. She decided to face these feelings and to try to understand where they came from and how to deal with them.

Her apprehension was triggered by uncertainty about the future. How much longer could she continue to entertain at home? How much longer would friends want to come to visit? How much longer could she continue to get away for a few hours by herself to meet friends or see a show? How much longer could she manage at home without help? Amanda no longer avoided these questions. They were reasonable, and the feelings of concern they generated provided the motivation for Amanda to become better informed about the nature and course of Bill's disorder and to begin formulating some tentative plans for the increasing amount of personal care he would inevitably require.

Her anger was harder for Amanda to accept, as it is for many people. We will deal with anger in detail in a later chapter. But Amanda knew she felt angry with Bill at times, and she no longer tried to pretend that her feelings for Bill were the same as before. She was through denying her feelings. She realized they didn't go away just because she closed her eyes to them. She had taken the first step. Now she was ready to reexamine her expectations of Bill, of herself, of others, and of life in general.

For you, the caregiver, examining your expectations represents the next step on the road to more effective coping. We hope you are ready to move on.

CHAPTER **3**

Expecting the Unexpected

Have you ever found yourself in a novel situation? One that was totally unfamiliar to you and that offered you no basis for predicting what might happen next? Perhaps it was a new job, a new neighborhood, or your first day in a new school or summer camp. You didn't know what to expect.

Part of the appeal of familiar surroundings lies in their predictability. We soon learn what to expect, and our expectations are usually confirmed. This goes for people, too.

The predictability of human behavior makes social interaction possible. We learn to expect people to behave in characteristic ways, and for the most part, they do.

In Alzheimer's disease, however, erratic behavior occurs without any apparent reason. Certainly you see no outward evidence of brain injury and no apparent physical defect. Yet your family member's behavior no longer conforms to your expectations. How do you feel? How can you restore and maintain your own sense of order in the face of chaotic behavior?

Joe Caravello's reactions were fairly typical. Since his retirement, Joe and his wife Maria had centered their lives around their family. Sunday and holiday dinners, with lots of good food for all the children and grandchildren, were traditional.

When Maria began forgetting to buy food for the family's Sunday dinners, when she forgot where the supermarket was, and when she hid Joe's glasses under the underwear in his dresser drawer, the family realized that something was very wrong. They started on the long road from family doctor, to neurologist, to neuropsychological evaluation, to brain scan, until a diagnosis of Alzheimer's disease was made.

The doctor explained that her condition, a dementing illness, was untreatable and progressively deteriorative, both mentally and physically. Changes in her brain would result in changes in her personality, her behavior and her physical functioning. While her life expectancy could be three years or fifteen years, the disease would ultimately be fatal.

But Maria continued to look like her old self most of the time. And she managed, with Joe's help and the help of the two older daughters, who came over from time to time, to continue functioning at home pretty well. Then one Sunday afternoon, in the middle of dinner, Maria stood up and told them all to go home. She said she didn't want to see them anymore. She was sick and tired of all of them.

Joe was mortified. The children were hurt. Joe told her to stop putting on an act. They knew she wasn't all that crazy.

They had heard the doctor explain that Alzheimer's disease was a dementing illness. But to them, the word "dementia" conjured up images of a crazy person, ill-kempt and unwashed, running around at night setting fire to the house. Maria was nothing like that. She looked very much like her old self, nice and neat, and if you weren't told of her mental lapses, you wouldn't know that anything much was wrong with her.

And yet, here she was, ordering her own children and grandchildren out of the house in the middle of their regular Sunday dinner. They were angry, hurt, bewildered, and outraged. Nothing in their experience prepared the Caravellos for Maria's outburst. In spite of her illness, they continued to expect what people learn to expect: socially appropriate behavior.

They had not yet learned step number one of dealing with a person with a dementing illness: Expect the unexpected. Expect demented behavior.

We know what to expect of a two-year-old child, of a five-year-old child, of a ten-year-old child. We expect a child to act childishly, each according to age-related appropriate behavior. We do not expect a two-year-old to read, nor do we ascribe his inability to read to willfulness, spite, or just plain bad manners. We know that his inability to read is a function of his immature brain. There are socially accepted norms of behavior for children, as there are for adults.

However, the socially approved rules of conduct for people in general do not apply to persons with dementing illness. The victims are losing their ability to conform to social norms. Expecting them to do so is as realistic as expecting the two-year-old to read. Or the paraplegic to walk. Or the blind to see. But expectations of people with brain failure cannot be so clearly delineated.

There is only one certainty: the patient will act dementedly.

But what is demented behavior? It has no rules, no descriptions, no guidelines. It violates all we have ever learned to expect of other people. Dementia, by definition, precludes predictability. It is behavior that is off balance, and it catches the family off balance. A person with a deteriorating brain will exhibit socially deteriorated behavior, regardless of how she looks today, or how she acted yesterday. You can predict socially unacceptable behavior, but you can't predict what form it will take, or when it will crop up.

When the norms of behavior are violated, one generally becomes angry. If you are standing in line at the movie theater and someone comes along and pushes his way up to the front of the line, you generally become upset. You say to yourself, "Some nerve. He shouldn't do that." Because the norm is quite clear: Wait your turn like the rest of us. But there are no norms for dementia. The only norm is demented behavior, that is, the bizarre, the socially unacceptable, and, sometimes, the destructive. The only realistic expectation is to expect the unexpected—the bizarre, the socially unacceptable, the destructive.

The bizarre behavior is not volitional. The demented person is a prisoner of her deteriorated brain.

Imagine how you would feel if you lost your cues for person or place. Suppose you suddenly found yourself bobbing about in mid-ocean, with no land in sight, no stars, no compass. You can't remember how you got there, or how long you were there. All your familiar cues for time and place suddenly vanished. How do you think you would feel? In all likelihood, you would feel confused about where you were, and who you were. You might even feel terrified. You might say strange things. You might do strange things.

To the person whose memory has become unreliable, the world may well look like a place without cues, a world without order or meaning. That person's mind is bobbing around in an empty sea. What may appear to you to be willful behavior may be the behavior of a mind that has lost its moorings.

Your family member is not being willful, or vicious, or purposely trying to frustrate you any more than a heart-attack victim is deliberately trying to frighten you—she is simply acting on the signals that her deteriorated brain is sending.

Learning to expect the unexpected is not easy. In fact, it's very difficult. One of the confounding factors is that in its early stages, the mental deterioration of the person with Alzheimer's disease is not unitary or consistent. He may dress himself one day, and then the next he might stare at his shirt without comprehension. He may arrange his tools in the workshed very neatly, yet not know what to do with his knife and fork. He may, like Steve Jenkins, ask you the same question fifteen times in the space of two minutes, and yet he may appear to function with apparent ease in social situations.

Ruth Jenkins believed that Steve had stabilized. He seemed to enjoy socializing with old friends, although he had trouble remembering names and sometimes was at a loss for a specific word. Ruth constantly had her radar out, ready to supply the name, the word, ready to cover up for him. No one knew that there was anything wrong with him. After all, don't we all get a little forgetful when we get older? Ruth was confident that with her help, Steve would continue to function in this way indefinitely. Then one evening, they had a few friends over for dinner. After the initial greetings and exchange of pleasantries, Steve asked Isabel Kaufman how their son Fred was doing at college. There was a shocked silence. Fred had been killed in an automobile accident about three months before. The Kaufmans, at the urging of their closest friends—including Ruth—had just begun to accept some social engagements.

Ruth was speechless. How could Steve have said a thing like that? He couldn't have forgotten, especially since they had attended the funeral. He couldn't have forgotten that!

The dinner party broke up early. Ruth was convinced that in some incomprehensible way, Steve had done this deliberately to upset her, to test her endurance, to ruin her dinner party. He could behave decently when he wanted to.

Because she had not accepted his inevitable decline, she tried to find a rational explanation for his irrational behavior. So, she reasoned, some old, long-suppressed "ornery" streak in him was surfacing. Everyone said that personality traits, especially the less-endearing ones, get exaggerated as people age. That notion sustained Ruth until the next time Steve misbehaved. Then she had to look at reality. She had to give up her expectation that he had remained and would remain relatively intact, with some occasional lapses, harking back to his old personality. She had to learn to expect demented behavior.

Just as the demented person has lost his moorings, so the caregiver, expecting sameness and continuity in human relations, responds with bewilderment and some degree of disorganization. The familiar responses are no longer there. The flow of the relationship has been disrupted, never to return to its former course.

Muriel Simpson's mother, Mrs. O'Connor, began to hide things. At first it was her toothbrush, then her coral beads, which the children had given her one Mother's Day. Then she hid money, and one day Muriel found a bunch of bananas stuffed away in a shoe box on top of a closet. At this, Muriel's pent-up rage with her mother exploded. Didn't she know that food will spoil, and that mold will grow, and bugs will come, and didn't she know perfectly well that no one is going to touch her things, and that no one wants her things?

Mrs. O'Connor remained unmoved. She was convinced that people came in during the night and stole her most prized possessions. No amount of persuasion could convince her otherwise. Muriel's distress became acute when her mother accused her of being the chief culprit. Muriel was "devastated." She always remembered her mother as a kind and gentle person. They had had a good relationship all their lives. How could her mother now accuse her of stealing her things— she, Muriel, who was the most devoted of her children?

Muriel expected kindness to be repaid with kindness, loving care to be repaid with appreciation. She didn't deserve this!

Muriel knew that her mother was suffering from a serious brain disease. What she still had not accepted was that changes in the brain cause changes in the personality, that the once gentle woman, whom she didn't hesitate to take into her house when her father died, could become the suspicious, accusatory woman who was now so difficult to live with. It took Muriel some time to realize that her mother was, literally, a different person. She was not, as some people said, a person in second childhood, but a demented adult, an adult whose illness severely limited her access to her lifetime store of knowledge and experience. Because of this, she had become a person whose day-to-day behavior had become unpredictable.

The person whose brain is failing is struggling against great odds to protect his badly bruised ego. The productive, communication and survival skills that he developed over the years and that had enabled him to function in society are now disintegrating. As he loses the ability to interact effectively with other people and with his environment, his powers to satisfy his own needs and wants decrease. As his powers decrease, his world constricts. His self-esteem diminishes.

The once independent head of a household has become a dependent person. The family nurturer must now be nurtured. Part of the person is sufficiently aware of his lowered status to be angry and resentful of it. To protect his fragile ego, he may lash out at you, the caregiver, and blame you for his present woes. He can't change. He acts compulsively out of the demands of his failing brain. Only you can change, by changing your expectation of him.

Sarah Gordon sometimes forgot what she had so painstakingly learned. She knew that Alzheimer patients sometimes wander away, sometimes become violent or abusive, and sometimes become so unmanageable that the family's survival seems at stake.

When he first came to live with her, Sarah's father was fairly helpful. He sometimes did the dishes, swept the terrace, and even went on errands if they were within walking distance. Then he began to refuse to help at all. He said that he was being abused and would call the police if such demands continued. He also began to leave heaps of crumbs and globs of spaghetti and sauce all around his dinner plate and on the floor. He refused to clean up after himself.

Sarah tried to accept this as an inevitable result of his illness. Then one day, he urinated in the waste-paper basket in the den. That was too much. Sarah lost control.

"What's wrong with you? Are you crazy? How can you do such a thing? I don't know what to do with you. You can't stay here if you act so crazy!"

Although Sarah's outburst was understandable, the result was that her father went into a state of intense agitation. He experienced a full fledged catastrophic reaction, a loss of control often seen in Alzheimer's patients. He shouted obscenities and attempted to flee the house. Finding the doors and windows locked, he tried to throw a chair through the glass. He was subdued only after the family physician arrived and administered a sedative.

While she thought that she had accepted her father's erratic behavior, Sarah was unprepared for a violation of what, to her, was a sacrosanct value of civilized life: hygiene. This was a transgression of the first order. Her reaction was commensurate with her evaluation of the misdeed.

Her father responded to bizarre signals in his head and acted bizarrely. Sarah responded to his bizarre behavior and acted overemotionally. The normal, expected behaviors by which she had ordered her life had given way to the fragmented, the disorderly, the unacceptable.

As the victim loses his mental anchors, it is important for you, the caregiver, to secure yours. That means anchoring yourself in reality. It means giving up your own ideas about how your parent or mate "should" be behaving. It means giving up your own maladaptive notions of how he should behave and accepting the reality of how he actually does behave.

It means giving up all of the dysfunctional self-statements that interfere with formulating more realistic expectations about your family member's behavior.

Let's review some of those dysfunctional self-statements and look at some better alternatives:

Instead of Saying . . .	Tell Yourself . . .
She looks fine, so she must be fine.	Outward appearance is not a good indicator of brain function.
Sometimes she does better in certain areas so she should always do better in those areas.	Demented behavior changes from day to day and from moment to moment.
He can do better when he wants to.	His lapses are due to brain changes, not lack of motivation.
His behavior should be consistent and predictable.	His behavior will be inconsistent and unpredictable.
He is just being stubborn, vindictive and uncooperative, just like he used to be.	His behavior may look like the surfacing of his old unpleasant traits. But when his brain changed, he changed.
He should continue to act as he has always acted in the past.	His behavior will change as his brain changes, whether I like it or not.
She is deliberately acting badly, just to get my goat.	She can no longer act purposefully. She has little control over her behavior. I can control mine.

Instead of Saying . . .	**Tell Yourself . . .**
He must never do this dreadful thing again.	There he goes again! He's done it before and in all likelihood he'll do it again, if not this, then something equally bad, or worse. I'll expect it and accept it. Then I can cope with it better.
She is in second childhood.	She is becoming a demented adult.

PART **II**

Taking Charge of Your Emotional Life

CHAPTER **4**

Your Feelings

Part II of this book deals with your feelings—how you generate them and how you can change them.

As a caregiver of an Alzheimer patient, you have sometimes been overwhelmed by negative emotions. The pain, sorrow, and frustration of seeing your close family member—your parent, or the person with whom you have shared your life—deteriorate to a point beyond recognition, places a tremendous burden upon your emotional resources. You have felt anger and shame. You have, at times, felt guilty about your actions or reactions. You have no doubt experienced self-pity. You've probably been depressed a good deal of the time. Often, you've become so frustrated that you wanted to scream. Sometimes you did.

Strong negative feelings can be very painful. They can also be distinctly maladaptive. They get in the way of finding better alternatives, both for yourself and for your sick relative. Strong negative feelings, while all too human and understandable, are generally not productive.

There are many shades and gradations of emotions. Take anger, for example. Try to visualize a continuum of emotion, with annoyance at one end, and rage at the other: annoyance . . . displeasure . . . irritation . . . anger . . . rage.

There is a whole range of possible emotional responses along the same dimension, varying in intensity. Obviously, the person in a state of rage has fewer adaptive choices available to him than the mildly angered or the annoyed.

You, the caregiver, have choices. You can choose to feel irritated, annoyed, or enraged when your family member acts in a manner you find difficult.

How, you ask, can I choose my emotional response? Don't my feelings arise spontaneously? Isn't that what's meant by a gut reaction? It may be your gut reaction, but your gut responds to what's in your head.

In this section, we will show you how to take charge of your emotional life. At any one moment, you may feel a whole constellation of emotions. Emotional responses are complex and not neatly sorted out. You may, for example, feel anger, self-pity, and frustration, all mixed up in one emotional outburst, or in one long, sustained emotional undertone to your life.

In order to help you apply the logic of emotions to your own situation, we will separate your complex emotional response into its identifiable emotional components and deal with each individually. In a series of conversations between ourselves, the authors, and you, the caregiver, we will show you how to identify the dysfunctional thoughts that generate your emotional upsets. We will show you how to challenge those thoughts, and how to replace them with messages and beliefs that are more attuned to reality and that offer better emotional and behavioral options.

We think that you will recognize the thoughts and

feelings expressed in these conversations. We hope that you will learn from them how to help yourself feel better and do better—for your Alzheimer relative, and for yourself.

CHAPTER 5

Anger: Sometimes I Get So Mad

I've been caring for my husband for a couple of years. I know that having a spouse with Alzheimer's disease is no bed of roses, and I try to do my best for him. But lately, it's been getting harder and harder, and I'm having trouble controlling my temper. I feel annoyed and irritated much of the time. Sometimes I get furious. He shows me no consideration, even though I do everything I can for him. His behavior is just outrageous. Last night he made me so mad, I threw a plate on the floor.

You just said some contradictory things. You said that you feel annoyed and irritated much of the time. Irritation and annoyance sound like quite appropriate responses to obnoxious behavior. After all, you can't be expected to be indifferent to behavior that violates the norms of social intercourse. But irritation and annoyance would not lead to the kind of emotional outburst that would result in your throwing a plate on the floor. Obviously, your fury with him caused you to do that. Tell us what occurred just before the outburst.

I had worked so hard to prepare one of his favorite dishes, and he acted like he didn't care. He complained about the taste. Then he wouldn't use his knife and fork. Instead, he dug in with his fingers. I really couldn't stand it—it was so disgusting. I patiently corrected him several times. I even got up and went over to show him what to do. But when I sat down, he just went back to using his fingers. I became enraged—that's when I threw the plate.

Can you recall what you were saying to yourself just before you threw the plate?

I felt that this was absolutely the last straw. I simply could not tolerate any more. I yelled, "How can you eat in that disgusting manner? That's revolting. Stop it." But he kept right on. He was like a stubborn child. That's when I saw red.

Then you told yourself—and him—that he must absolutely not behave in this obnoxious way? In other words, that he must absolutely not behave like a person with a brain disorder. Now I ask you: Why should a person with a brain disorder act like one with an intact brain? It would certainly be fine if he could, but if he could, you wouldn't be taking care of him. He would be taking care of himself. In other words, your perception of him is not quite realistic. That's why you became so enraged. You think that he "should" have the table manners of a normal person. Where is the evidence that this is possible?

No place. I know that he has a brain disorder. But when I get angry like that, what am I supposed to do? Pretend that all is sweetness and light? Hold it in? Isn't it better to release it in some way?

You did release it, by throwing the plate. How did you feel just after you did that? Did you feel better?

Yes and no. I calmed down, but I felt that I lost control. I felt justified, in a way, but I also felt ashamed and sorry. But would I have felt better if I had kept my anger in? Pretend I didn't feel it?

Many people believe that there are only two ways to deal with anger. One is to deny your feeling, keep it in, play a constant charade with yourself. The other is to give vent to your feeling, to get rid of it by letting it out. Both are maladaptive.

Denial of feelings constricts and blunts your emotional life. It creates a situation in which you label feelings as good or bad. And then you say, "I mustn't have bad feelings like anger." And so you repress your anger. But you haven't fooled yourself. You know you feel it, and so you may even decide that you are a bad person for having the bad feelings that you are ashamed of. This could have serious emotional consequences for yourself.

Another alternative is to express your anger. You might tell someone off, or break dishes, or punch pillows. If the person you are telling off is your husband with Alzheimer's disease, the chances are that he won't understand the cause of your fury, will feel attacked, and will react with even worse behavior. And it's most unlikely that he will stop the obnoxious behavior that precipitated your anger in the first place. If the dishes you break are your own, that's O.K., providing they aren't your grandmother's heirloom china; if it's in someone else's house or in a restaurant, the consequences might be quite unpleasant. If punching pillows is your favorite outlet, it doesn't hurt anyone and may even help you let off steam. But there aren't always pillows left handily around whenever, and wherever, your anger mounts. By the time you find one, you may either have cooled off, screamed at your husband, or broken some more dishes.

Then you give me no choice. I'm trapped between a rock and a hard place.

Not exactly. There is a third choice. That is, not to feel all that angry.

But my feelings are my feelings. I don't manufacture them. They happen.

You create them by what you say about the situation. And you can change them by changing what you say about the situation. Let's go back to what you said before. You told yourself that he must not behave like a person with a dementing illness. In saying that, you are making a demand that your husband behave in a manner in which he is not capable of behaving. If that were possible, that would spare you and him much grief. But can he? Obviously not.

Then what am I supposed to do? Like what's happening?

No. That would be neither appropriate nor possible. But between liking it, and becoming infuriated by it, there is a whole gamut of emotional responses available to you, depending upon what you say to yourself about it.

Like what?

To wish that this were not happening is entirely reasonable. To demand it is irrational. And so, when you say, either to yourself or to him, "This must not be," you are making a demand based on irrational premises.

If you wished that this were not happening, you would undoubtedly have felt appropriately annoyed or irritated at his behavior. Since you demanded that this were not happening, you became infuriated and lashed out.

Then are you saying that the next time that he acts disagreeably or stubbornly, or even disgustingly, all I have to do is to say to myself, "I wish he weren't acting so badly," and let it go at that? And then I won't feel angry?

Yes and no! It's not easy, in the face of what may look like provocation, to change your evaluation of the situation. It takes continual rehearsal to replace the maladaptive "shoulds" and "musts" with the more adaptive "I wish" and "I prefer." It is necessary to say "I wish" and "I prefer" over and over again until these words become not just semantic change, that is, not just a way of saying, but cognitive change, a way of believing. If you just say it once or twice, and let it go at that, you will not make this new way a part of your response repertory. Say it, rehearse it, believe it, until it becomes an automatic response. That takes a great deal of effort.

Suppose I say it over and over, and then he makes me mad again. Then what?

Let's look at your remark, "He made me so mad . . ." That's a pretty loaded statement. That assumes that he is responsible for your emotions, that he has the power to determine your responses. Is he pulling your strings, or are you an autonomous person, capable of taking charge of your own emotional life?

Are you telling me that his behavior has absolutely nothing to do with my response?

No. His behavior is the trigger, or the stimulus. You can't control that. Your emotions are the response. Between the stimulus, his behavior, and the response, your anger, are the beliefs that are in your head. That is where you can exercise choice. And in exercising choice concerning your beliefs about what's happening, you determine your emotional response. You can do that by vigorously practicing a different set of self-statements. Like saying, "I wish he didn't do that," instead of "It's awful if he does that."

All right, so I practice saying "I wish he didn't behave in this manner," instead of "He mustn't behave in this manner." What else?

The next time he behaves in a manner that you find difficult or "uncivilized" say to yourself, "There he goes again." That may not sound like much, but it is actually saying, "He's acting in a manner that I have every reason to expect. He is suffering from a dementing illness, and therefore he is acting dementedly." If you expect him to act dementedly, and he does, then your expectation is fulfilled. You won't be taken by surprise. You are less likely to feel anger.

Reminding yourself to be realistic in your expectations will help you to accept what you don't like, such as eating with his fingers and complaining about the food you so laboriously—and lovingly—prepared. You will even not be too upset by the fact that he no longer appreciates what you do for him.

Yes, that also made me furious. I try so hard for him, and all I get is either indifference or abuse.

Again, there is a "should" there. It sounds like you're saying, "He should appreciate me and my efforts and it's awful and terrible if he doesn't." He doesn't appreciate you, because that takes more cognitive ability—brain power—than he now has. When you understand and accept that, you will no longer respond with anger and hurt at his seeming indifference.

Sometimes, his stubbornness gets my goat. Last night, he absolutely refused to take his clothes off at bedtime. That made me so mad, I was at my wit's end.

Suppose you restate the problem as follows: He became very stubborn and refused to take his clothes off at bedtime. I became very angry about that.

If you state it in that fashion, you will see that the second part, "I became very angry about that," is not a necessary or even logical consequence of the first. Again, his refusal to take his clothes off was his behavior, your anger was your emotional response to a situation beyond your control. His bizarre behavior was the result of his illness. Your anger was the result of your illogical expectation that he "should"—like all normal people—take his clothes off at bedtime. Why should he?

Obviously, because it's better for him to sleep in night clothes than in street clothes.

You are assuming that he must do that which is better for him. And you are saying that if he doesn't, then you will upset yourself unduly.

What if it's something important? What if he refuses to take his pills?

Let's separate those acts that are probably in his best interest, and those emotional responses that are in your best interest. If he refuses to cooperate in some act that is important, such as taking his medicine, in what way does your charged emotional response, which we call anger, help to overcome his resistance? Or help you to accept the fact that he won't do the thing that is best for him?

Actually, no way.

Then suppose that you try something else. Suppose that you say to yourself, "I have offered him his medicine (or tried to undress him for bed). If he refuses it, it's not the end of the world. I'll try again later. Or, if worse comes to worst, he'll skip his medicine this time, or he'll sleep in his clothes tonight. And I don't have to upset myself that much about it."

But must I always let him have his way? Like a spoiled child?

It is inappropriate to view a demented adult as if he were a spoiled child. Your husband is not in the same situation as a child who has not yet learned the limits of acceptable social behavior and who is still assimilating new experiences in order to make organized sense out of the world. Your husband is in the process of losing his ability to understand the world, or what is expected of him in everyday situations. He is losing access to the accumulated experiences of his life stored in memory and his ability to relate new information to that memory storage. He is in the process of losing touch with cues to time or place, to the identity of other people, and eventually to his own identity. All this renders him confused and highly dependent upon you for his survival. But this is not like the dependency of a young child on his parents. The child's dependency is temporary, your husband's is not. The child's view of the world is expanding, your husband's is contracting.

When he acts stubbornly, he is, in a way, saying, "I am not a child. Don't treat me like one. I am still an autonomous person, and you can't make me do what I don't want to do."

Now, if you want to make yourself furious about that, that is your privilege. But you don't have to. Isn't it more adaptive to accept his refusal, saying to yourself, "He is acting dementedly, not childishly. That is the only way he knows how to act. I don't have to be angry about that, although I'm certainly annoyed."

But sometimes he's disgusting, like when he slops his food all over the table, and he won't stop.

Now you are confusing his behavior with his personhood. Let us explain. Every person has a whole array of traits—good and bad, adaptive and non-adaptive. All these traits, taken together, describe the person. No single one defines him.

When you say, "He's disgusting," you are defining him by a single behavior that you understandably find objectionable. But is that all of him? Hardly.

It would be more appropriate to say, "Sometimes he does things that I find disgusting." In this way, you define your own response to the act—an admittedly disgusting act—without labeling the person as a disgusting person. When you separate the act, your response to it, and the person who committed it, you will find his behavior easier to tolerate. And you will undoubtedly feel less anger toward the person.

What about when he makes ridiculous accusations against me? Like saying I stole his hairbrush or his watch? I try to reason with him and point out how absurd this is. And when I think that I've gotten through to him, he starts all over again. That's when I lose my temper.

You think that you are speaking to a person who can benefit from your reasoned and reasonable arguments. But you aren't. If he were not demented, he would not make those irrational accusations. He doesn't remember where his hairbrush or watch are. So to protect himself and his own fragile ego, he makes the accusation that you hid them from him.

So you see, your anger, while directed toward him, is really generated by your unrealistic expectations of him.

Sometimes I feel anger, not because of anything specific that he does, but because of what he has done to my life.

This is the most difficult problem to deal with. It is probably the underlying cause of most of your resentment, because your life has indeed been unalterably changed in ways you never anticipated by his illness. But did he do it? Or is it something that happened to him, as well as to you? Totally outside of his volition? And his control? Isn't this his unfortunate reality, as well as yours?

This is a problem that we will have to return to over and over again in the course of these discussions. It is one that we will have to examine in its many ramifications, as we disentangle the many overlapping disabling emotions that now beset you.

While it is human to get angry, it is unproductive to stay angry. We exhaust ourselves and alienate others. Since anger is largely generated by our insistence that the world and its inhabitants conform to our demands, we can damp down our anger by giving up these unrealistic demands. We can still try to accomplish our goals to the best of our ability, but we don't have to get furious if things don't work out as we wanted, or if others don't act as we think they should.

Ask yourself: Does your anger facilitate or impede your making more adaptive decisions, or finding some better solutions for a difficult situation?

If it doesn't help you, then why not stubbornly refuse to enrage yourself?

Here are some suggestions:

Instead of Saying . . .	Tell Yourself . . .
She absolutely mustn't do that.	I would prefer that she not do that, but she might anyway.
I demand that she stop that.	She will not necessarily do what I demand. (If it is something dangerous, then naturally, I will have to find the way, without anger, to stop it.)
She must do what's best for her.	It would be preferable if she does what's best for her. But if she doesn't, it's too bad, but not terrible.
Sometimes she is disgusting.	Sometimes she does things that I find disgusting.
She does things just to be ornery.	She does what her deteriorated brain tells her to do.

Instead of Saying . . .	**Tell Yourself . . .**
She is driving me crazy.	I am driving myself crazy about what she does. She can't change, but I can.
She acts like a spoiled child.	She acts like a demented adult.
She ruined my life.	My life has been changed as a result of her illness. So has hers. That's our reality.

CHAPTER 6

Shame: I Feel Mortified

About a year ago, my mother came to live with me. She had been living alone, and life became more and more difficult for her. She lost things. She forgot people and places. She had occasional periods of disorganization. She needed help dressing and running her household. So I asked her to come and live with me. It wasn't easy, but I managed.

Last week, I helped Mom to bed. Then I had some friends in for an evening of bridge. At about 9:30, Mom appeared in the living room, in her thin nightgown, without her robe, unkempt, her dentures not in her mouth, speaking incoherently.

I tried to get her back to bed, but she refused to budge. She mumbled in an agitated manner, and the best I could make out was that "they" were in her room and had stolen her dentures.

I tried, as calmly as I could, to explain to her that no one would want her dentures—they were made to fit her and were of no use to anyone else. She shouted "Are you telling me I'm crazy? I saw them take them."

Then I remembered that the doctor had given me a mild sedative to use if she needed it. I gave her the sedative, and after a while she calmed down and went back to bed.

The whole episode took about a half hour. I was mortified.

What were you mortified about?

The evening was ruined. My friends looked badly shaken, although they tried to pretend that they understood. I couldn't look them in the face.

What went through your mind?

I was ashamed.

Of what?

I was ashamed of my mother's behavior. I felt disgraced. I was angry because she ruined my evening.

Let's take this one step at a time. You were ashamed of your mother's behavior. Are you responsible for your mother's behavior?

No.

Can you control her behavior?

No.

Do you feel that your mother can control her behavior?

No.

Do you think that your mother was ashamed of her behavior?

No. She was totally unaware of what she was doing. I'm sure that she forgot the whole episode immediately.

Then you took upon yourself the "obligation" of being ashamed of behavior for which you are not responsible, that you cannot control, that the person who committed the offensive acts cannot control, and for which she is not ashamed. Isn't that taking a big load upon yourself?

I guess so. That's how I felt.

Let's read the Merriam-Webster Dictionary (1974) definition of shame: "A painful sense of having done something wrong, improper or immodest." Do you think that you did something wrong, improper, or immodest?

Yes, I did something wrong. I shouldn't have invited friends over to my house as long as my mother lives with me.

Has she ever displayed such disordered behavior before?

No, she's been peculiar, but never obnoxious.

Then are you saying that you should have been able to predict this?

In a way, yes. I know that AD is a deteriorative disease. I've read enough about this to know that people with this disease often act in thoroughly unacceptable ways. I just refused to face the fact that she would come to this. It's so unlike her.

It's true that, in dealing with an AD victim, one of the most important changes in one's own thinking is to give up expecting the patient's behavior to follow a predictable course. The patient's behavior generally violates everything you have ever learned about social intercourse. The best prediction you can make is to expect the unexpected. But you haven't learned that yet. It's difficult because it means unlearning previous expectations of human behavior, based upon a lifetime of experience, and substituting new expectations for which your experience has not prepared you.

But she has, in fact, acted peculiarly, although not so outrageously, in the past. So I think it was wrong to have exposed other people to this traumatic situation.

Undoubtedly, most people prefer to distance themselves from behavior that they can't understand and that is outside of their experience. That's one of the problems that leads to the social isolation of families of AD victims. That's reality. When you recognize and accept that reality, you can begin to make some adjustments to continue to have as full a social life as possible under the circumstances. However, when you say that you did something "wrong" by inviting your friends in for an evening of bridge, you are invoking a moral judgment upon yourself. And you punish yourself with feelings of humiliation.

I don't feel responsible for my mother's behavior, but I did, indeed, feel humiliated by it. How could I not?

Are you confusing your mother's behavior with your own? She is the one who committed the asocial acts. Not you.

Yes, but isn't there a sense of identification with a parent that starts in childhood and is carried over into adulthood?

Often there is. Let's look at that. How is it relevant to your feeling of shame and humiliation now?

I remember, when I was young, I always had a feeling of pride that my mother was so pretty and well groomed and well spoken and that people liked her. That made me feel good about myself. And now . . .

Yes, children often do derive status from their parents—their appearance, their social and financial positions, their lifestyles. But as an adult, when you

have made your own way in the world, do you feel
that your mother's deterioration, in some way, reflects
upon you?

It doesn't make sense to think that, but I do feel demeaned by my
mother's behavior.

Let's imagine that you were sitting in the living
room, reading a book, and your mother wandered in,
in her nightgown, disheveled, without her teeth, mum-
bling incoherently. Would you have felt ashamed or
humiliated by her behavior?

No.

What do you think you would have felt?

I would probably have felt angry, or annoyed, or bewildered, but
not shame.

Then what else do you think you said to yourself
that evening, when your friends were there? Something that made the difference to you between feeling
anger, annoyance, and bewilderment on the one hand,
and shame and humiliation on the other?

I said to myself, "What will they think of me?"

Not, "What will they think of Mom?" but "What
will they think of me?"

Yes.

So, are you still identifying with your parent, as if
your status is still derived from her?

That may be so.

Then how can you change that?

By telling myself that I'm an independent and separate person, and I'm not responsible for my mother's behavior.

Yes, and at the same time, it would be wise to examine the question, "What will they think of me?" Regardless of what they actually think of you, suppose you ask yourself, "What difference does their opinion of me make?" Does their opinion of you shape you? Make you into a person you are not?

Aren't we all influenced by what people think of us?

Yes, we are, to a great degree. But even more, we are influenced by what we *think* that people think of us. For example, you felt humiliated by what you thought people thought of you. Do you really know what they thought? Did you ask them? Or did you infer what they thought, by projecting your own self-imposed feeling of humiliation upon them?

No, of course I didn't ask them. I assumed they would be embarrassed and that they would think less of me because of my mother's behavior.

And suppose they actually did think less of you because of it. Whose problem would that be?

Theirs, now that you put it that way. In the future, when my mother acts up in front of other people, I can just tell myself that if other people think less of me because of it, that's their problem.

Yes. And if you had not felt shame and embarrassment, what do you think you could have said to your friends that night?

I could simply have said, "My mother is sick. She has AD. I'm sorry to have to interrupt the game, but I have to take care of her now."

That would have been an honest and open way of dealing with the situation without embarrassment or shame.

So you see, that feeling of shame and humiliation actually prevented you from handling the situation in a more appropriate way.

Fear of what other people think can become a prison that shuts you off from creative thinking and flexible behaviors. Shame is often the key that locks the prison door.

———— • ————

Next week, we will have the annual office party. Everyone brings a mate or a date. I'll go alone.

Helen used to enjoy these parties, and I always enjoyed them, too. Last year, when I came without her, I told everyone that she was down with the flu. Then during the year, when groups of friends went bowling, I said that Helen couldn't join us because of her back problem. I went alone. I don't know what to tell people next week.

What is Helen's problem? Why can't she attend your parties?

She has AD.

Why can't you say that?

Tell people that she's demented? Most people, by now, have seen TV programs about senile dementia—about how people slowly lose their minds and can't speak and become incontinent. I can't tell people that that's what's wrong with Helen.

Why not?

Because I'd be ashamed to.

Suppose that she had a heart problem and couldn't go out much. What would you tell people?

I'd tell them that she has a heart problem.

So you put AD in a separate class, different from other diseases that you can acknowledge. What's so different about it, that you put it in the closet?

Well, AD is a mental disorder. People who have it act peculiar or crazy.

And if they do—as indeed they do—why can't you acknowledge that?

Because when people hear that it's a mental disorder, they either become frightened, or they think it's funny. Sometimes they laugh when they hear an anecdote about some of the crazy things that somebody's elderly relative did. You know, there's always this image of elderly people as doddering old fools. Helen is not that old—she's sixty-one. But still, I feel ashamed. I hate to admit that she's like that.

Not taking Helen to social functions is entirely understandable. Change, large numbers of people, noise, and excitement are very disorganizing for AD patients. They are generally more comfortable with sameness and quiet, where they don't have to organize new and excessive stimuli into meaningful data. But what is so shameful about acknowledging that she has AD?

Because it is a disease associated with old age.

And what is shameful about old age?

I think that if people know that Helen has AD, they will look at me as if I'm over the hill. I still feel vigorous. I look pretty good for my age—I'm sixty-three—and I'm afraid that people will think of me as "that old man." That frightens me.

If people think of you as "that old man," does that make you an old man?

No, not really. But I would feel like one.

Then are you saying that if you told people that Helen has heart disease, you would not feel like an old man, but if you tell them that she has AD, then you will feel old?

That sounds foolish, doesn't it?

Not foolish. But not realistic either. You are projecting an image of yourself that is not based upon your own state of health and vigor, but upon a fear of what other people will think of you when they find out the true nature of your wife's illness.

And suppose that other people—I assume that you are thinking of the people in your office, many of whom may be quite young—do, in fact, think that you are over the hill. Does that put you over the hill?

No, it doesn't put me there, but it may tell me that I'm getting there.

And so, your problem is that Helen's disease—or a public acknowledgement of it—forces you to face your own aging. And why is aging shameful?

Aging itself isn't shameful. It's the decrepitude that comes with age that I feel is shameful. And Helen's illness is a sign that points in that direction. That's why I hate to tell people what she's suffering from.

There are two aspects of what you just said. In the first place, Alzheimer's disease—or what you call the decrepitude of old age—is not the inevitable accompaniment of aging that people once thought it was. That may have been true in Shakespeare's day, when people's lives ended in "Second childishness and mere oblivion / Sans teeth, sans eyes, sans taste, sans everything." Today, people are living longer, healthier lives than ever before. Many people continue to be active and productive into very advanced years. We cannot predict who will decline early and who will not, any more than we can predict who will perish in the next airplane accident. So we live with an uncertainty that permeates all life.

In the second place, while everyone would like to perpetuate youthful vigor, do you think that your worth as a person depends upon it?

I don't know. We live in a very youth-oriented society. And society certainly seems to devalue older people. Look at movies and television. You don't see too many old people portrayed.

That's true. But it's also true that there are big changes taking place. More and more movie stars are continuing to play important and interesting roles well into their advanced years. Your problem is partly that you, like many others, have bought the old stereotypes that old age is a disgrace and that old people must be hidden under a bushel.

So what shall I do about the office party?

Tell everyone that Helen can't come because she has Alzheimer's disease. Say it without apologies in your voice.

When you bring Helen's illness out of the closet,

you will feel much more comfortable about her and about yourself. The closet can be a stifling place to lock yourself into.

And remember, Alzheimer's is a disease, not a disgrace.

———————

We are three generations living together under one roof: my father-in-law, my fifteen-year-old daughter, seventeen-year-old son, my husband, and myself. My husband and I cope very well with my father-in-law, even though he does weird things sometimes. But the problem is the children. We have a nice house in a good neighborhood, with a recreation room for the children and their friends to hang out in. We've always tried to provide a welcome place so that they won't want to hang around places we might not approve of, and so we would know where they are.

For the past year, the children haven't brought their friends here. They make all sorts of excuses about why they must always go to other kids' homes on weekends.

We recently learned from my son that the problem is Grandpa. Grandpa sometimes wears his old sweater backward and insists on keeping it that way; he won't always let us shave him when he needs it; he is sometimes disheveled and needs a haircut; and, worst of all, occasionally when the children do have a party in the rec room, he has barged in and shouted at them to stop the racket. So the children simply moved their social lives away from home. We are very upset about that.

I'm sure that most parents prefer to have their teenagers socialize at home. Have you spoken to both of them about this?

Yes, and they've confessed that they are ashamed of Grandpa and don't want to face their friends when he is around.

Have you discussed the nature of his illness with them?

No.

Why not?

We didn't want to burden them with the knowledge that he's going to get worse.

Don't you think that ignorance is a greater burden for them?

We didn't realize that. We thought we could just ignore it. After all, Grandpa has been with us since they were very small. So we thought that they would just accept him as he grew older. As we do.

Put yourselves in their place. Their grandfather acts in a distinctly nonsocial or antisocial manner. No one has told them that he is sick and that his sickness has a name—Alzheimer's disease. No one has told them what to expect. And no one has prepared them for how to deal with this in front of their friends. So, to avoid what is, to them, a humiliating situation, they simply meet their friends elsewhere.

Perhaps you felt too ashamed of his deteriorating behavior to discuss it with them.

Maybe so. Maybe we covered our own feelings of shame by not leveling with them. Or maybe we didn't have enough confidence in our children to explain things properly to them.

Do you feel confident enough in your own acceptance of your father-in-law's condition to sit down with your children and explain the nature of the disease to them?

If you do, then you might also share with them the fact that his illness is very difficult for you, too, and that some of your own friendships have become strained because of it. So you understand why their friends are uncomfortable in Grandpa's presence. Urge them to explain to their friends that Grandpa is sick, and that's why he behaves so strangely.

At the same time, promise them that when they have friends over, you will always be home to keep an eye on Grandpa, so he will stay out of their way.

———•·•———

I generally take Ed out shopping with me. He likes to put packages into the cart and to push it while I look around. Sometimes he puts things in that I don't need, but that's O.K. I take them out a few minutes later. He likes the outings with me.

But yesterday, while we were going to the car after we made our purchases, he suddenly stood still and said he had to urinate. I told him that we're almost at the car, and that I would get him home as fast as I could. Then, without warning, a stream of urine ran down from his pants leg and onto the street. Some people stopped, stared at him, looked at me, and then pretended not to see.

You can imagine how embarrassed I felt.

What was so embarrassing?

Seeing this grown man wetting himself in the street like a child.

Do you think that he did it deliberately?

No, I'm sure he didn't. But he might have tried harder to control himself.

He might have. But do you think that he could have?

Well, he probably couldn't. But I don't think he even tried.

Are you saying that he should have behaved like a healthy person? One who has control over his bodily functions?

No, but I would certainly hope that he would try not to urinate in the street.

One could hope that. But what you are really saying is that a person with AD should behave like a person without AD. That doesn't sound very logical, does it? If he didn't have AD, he wouldn't be your dependent.

Yes, he's my dependent, and I do my best for him, but I don't like him to embarrass me by urinating in the street.

Let's separate what you just said into three parts and examine each statement separately.

He urinated in the street. That is a statement of fact. We think that you agree that he is losing control of his bodily functions. That is the result of his illness. Difficult as it is, that is something that you had better expect and accept.

I don't like it. There's no reason to like it. In fact, there's every reason to dislike it. However, since his bladder control is Ed's function, not yours, there is no way that you can change it. Lack of bladder control may seem childlike behavior, but he is not a child. A child can be toilet trained; Ed cannot. A child is learning new forms of behavior; your husband is losing his learned behaviors. A child's brain—which signals bodily activity—is flexible, open to new learning; Ed's brain is deteriorated, and therefore his behavior is rigid.

I am embarrassed by it. This is your emotional response to a very trying situation. Since this is your response, this is the part you can change.

How can I change that? Anyone would be embarrassed by that.

Most people would be. But they don't have to be. Not if they learn to apply the logic of feelings to their own distress.

How?

If you look at the statements "He urinated in the street" and "I was embarrassed," you will see that the first didn't cause your embarrassment. Rather, it triggered a chain of events that resulted in your embarrassment.

What kind of events? Nothing else happened.

What happened next was your evaluation of what he did. You didn't just stand there like a lamppost. Thoughts went through your mind. You made judgments. You said something to yourself about it. Do you know what these self-statements were?

No, I don't.

Just think for a moment. You just said that he behaved like a child. But you would not have been embarrassed if a child had done that. So you evaluated his behavior quite differently from the way you would have evaluated a child's behavior. You know that a child wets himself—and that's acceptable, even if inconvenient or annoying. But about Ed, you undoubtedly told yourself, "He shouldn't have done that. It's awful. What will people think? What will people think of me?" And that's why you were embarrassed.

That is the logic of feelings—that they result not from the event, but from your perception of the event. And while you can't change the event, you can change your perception of it.

How? My thoughts are my thoughts. They just come.

Yes, up to a point, they do. That's because you're used to thinking in a certain way. Like most people, you are used to thinking in "should nots" and "must nots"—"He should not do that" or "He must not do that," and you "awfulize"—"It's awful and terrible if he does that."

"Should nots" and "must nots" are demands that you make. And since they are absolute demands, you upset yourself if they are not met. And they are generally irrational. It's like saying, "It must not rain tomorrow." It is most unlikely that your demand will stop the rain from falling. But if you insist upon it, you will be most upset if the skies don't take heed. However, if you change that demand to a wish—"I wish that it won't rain tomorrow," or a preference—"I prefer that it doesn't rain tomorrow," then you have brought the ball back to your own court. That's realistic. Reality may be harsh, but in the long run, that's what you have to cope with.

And so, the next time that Ed does something asocial—as he will—instead of saying "He embarrassed me," say to yourself, "I wish he wouldn't do that." And stubbornly refuse to allow yourself to be embarrassed by it.

And remember, he didn't embarrass you. You embarrassed yourself by what you said about it.

Does that mean that if I give up the "must nots" and "should nots" about Ed's behavior, I will never be upset about what he does?

Not at all. It does mean that if you state a preference or wish, instead of a demand, you will undoubtedly feel annoyance or displeasure, instead of shame or embarrassment. And then you will find some more adaptive solutions to your problems.

Try it and see.

Instead of Saying . . .	**Tell Yourself . . .**
She humiliates me.	She acts dementedly. I am not responsible for that.
I feel mortified by her outrageous behavior.	I don't like her outrageous behavior, but I can't change it.
I know that she can behave better because sometimes she does.	Her behavior fluctuates. That's the way her brain works. I had better expect that.
I feel embarrassed just to tell people that my wife has Alzheimer's. What will they think?	What they think is their problem.
I feel ashamed of her demented behavior.	AD is a disease, not a disgrace. If I truly believe this, then I will not be ashamed of her behavior, any more than I would be ashamed of the seizures in epilepsy or the incoordination of multiple sclerosis.

CHAPTER **7**

Self-Pity: Poor Me

The other day, I prepared a delicious dinner—veal stew with onions, carrots, and all the really good seasonings that my mother loves. When it was ready, I went out onto the porch where I left Mom sitting and watching TV, to bring her in to dinner. She wasn't there. I looked all over the house, called her name. She was nowhere to be found. I got scared. I ran out into the street. I saw her slowly plodding along at the far end of the block. I grabbed my coat and ran after her. When I reached her, she was confused and frightened. She didn't know where she was. I slowly walked her home. When I came back, clouds of smoke were billowing from my pot of stew. The stew was ruined. So was the pot. I was furious! I just sat down and cried.

What did you cry about?

I cried about the ruined dinner. I cried for my mother. But mostly I cried for myself.

How did you feel?

I was furious. And I felt frustrated. I felt that Mom did me in. I know that she didn't do anything intentionally. That is, I know that now, with hindsight. But at the moment, that's how I felt. I do everything I can to make her comfortable. Then nothing turns out right. And I feel so frustrated.

So you felt a whole gamut of emotions, including frustration, anger, and mostly self-pity?

Yes, I suppose I did feel sorry for myself. And I do feel sorry for myself a good deal of the time. It's just too much! So every once in a while, I have a good cry. Is there anything wrong with that?

There's nothing wrong with crying. In fact, it's difficult to see how you could care for a dementing relative without shedding some tears. To feel sorry for yourself at times is human. The problem is *staying* sorry for yourself as a chronic condition. There are no rules telling people how they are supposed to react emotionally. There are no rights and wrongs about feelings. But some emotions, like self-pity, are debilitating.

What do you mean?

How did feeling sorry for yourself help you to deal with the burned pot, the ruined supper, and your mother's safety?

Obviously, it didn't. I didn't deal with any of them very well. I left the pot on the stove and gave Mom a peanut butter sandwich. I remember feeling as burnt out as the stew. Even trying to decide what to eat was too much for me, so I didn't eat anything.

Then the self-pity actually sapped your strength and reduced your motivation or ability to act.

That's true. But I can't help how I feel, can I?

Not so. How you feel in any situation depends largely on how you view it. What did you say to yourself about the incident? Just go back to that day and try to recollect.

I said "I've had it! I can't stand this much longer. This is too much for me."

Your situation certainly is tough! And it taxes you almost to the limit. But "almost" isn't total, is it?

No, but sometimes—like that day—I feel like I'm at the breaking point.

And that's when you say "I can't stand it any longer." Right?

Yes.

This is what we call "poor me" thinking. It blinds you to a very important fact: You *are* standing it. You could stand it even better if you change some of the things you are telling yourself about your situation.

How can I change my situation by telling myself different things?

What you say can't change your situation. But you can change how you feel about it.

How?

What you say represents your evaluation of your situation. It's how you perceive your life. And that determines how you feel and how you act.

You mean that I should just shut up, stop complaining, and make believe it doesn't bother me? Are there magic words that can make me happy?

No. We don't suggest that you stifle or deny your emotions. We do suggest that you can change them when it is in your own best interest to do so. Nor do we believe there are any magic words, any way we know that can make you happy while your mother is suffering from this serious deteriorating disease and you are called upon to take care of her. But there is a difference between feeling sad about a family tragedy and getting stuck in self-pity. Sadness is an appropriate reaction and unavoidable in your circumstances. Self-pity is debilitating and can be changed. It is the difference between saying "I can't stand it" and telling yourself "I don't like it, but it's what I've got, and I am standing it to the best of my ability."

When you say "I can't stand it," you feel quite miserable, and often make coping much more difficult. When you say "I don't like it but I can stand it, and, in fact, I am standing it," you ease your emotional burden. You stop feeling so sorry for yourself. Then you can seek ways to make your situation more tolerable.

I still don't see what's wrong with feeling sorry for myself, because things haven't worked out for me.

Because self-pity is an overreaction. It doesn't help you, and, as we have seen, it makes things worse for you. It's a way of saying "I must have what I want when I want, and if I don't get what I want, I must make myself entirely miserable." It would be nice to have what you want, but *must* you get it?

No.

Then why add self-pity to your already difficult life? Self-pity makes it more difficult to see your options.

What options? I don't see that I have any. I thought that my mothering days were over. Now I have to be a mother to my mother. That's not what I envisioned for myself when my children were growing up.

It's true that roles are often reversed as we get older. Children were nurtured by mother, from infancy to adulthood. And in middle age, they are often called upon to become the nurturers of dependent parents. That's part of the rhythm of life.

I understand. I have always known that. But I didn't expect it to happen to me. My mother always seemed so strong. She was the person who was always there for everyone. She was the emotional and physical prop for everyone. I guess I expected that it would always be that way. I am not asking to turn my back on my obligations to my mother. I just think that there must be ways of making it easier.

There are. Right now, we are not discussing practical measures, like getting some help, either on a daily or a part-time basis. Nor are we talking about the valid alternative of nursing-home placement. This may come in time. Now we are looking at cognitive and emotional alternatives.

What do you mean?

Cognitive means what your thoughts are, how you view what's happening and what you say to yourself about your situation. This affects your emotions, how you feel.

In what way?

If you say that it's terrible and awful that your mother's illness places this burden upon you, then you will feel pretty angry, frustrated, and self-pitying. If you tell yourself that this is not what you had hoped for but nevertheless what you've got, you will feel disappointed. Disappointment is a more adaptive response than anger, frustration, or self-pity because it does not lead to loss of motivation or self-defeating behavior. You can change how you think and how you feel, but it takes a good deal of effort.

Why should I work so hard to change my thoughts or my feelings?

Because that's what you *can* change. You can't make your mother whole again.

Well, it's not fair. And nothing that I tell myself can make me believe that it's fair, or ever will be fair.

No, it's not fair. And it never will be fair. Are you saying that it *should* be?

Why not?

Because fair for your mother is to have a daughter care for her in her hour of need. Fair for you is to have a mother who doesn't need your care. Fair for a drought-stricken farmer is to have rain. Fair for a family going on a long-planned vacation is to have continued sunshine. Fair for one is often not fair for another.

Yes, I know. But there was so much that I had planned for this time of my life, after all I went through with Henry's stroke, and then his death. After he died, I thought I would travel. I saved some money. The children are grown and on their way. I didn't expect this. I feel trapped.

Yes, in a sense you are trapped. Your situation represents a rotten outcome for yourself and for your mother. There is no way to get around this unfortunate truth, which is the ultimate source of much of your emotional turmoil. We alluded to it earlier, and we'll refer to it again throughout these talks: You never expected or planned for this. You didn't ask for it and you hate it. It prevents you from realizing your own hopes and dreams. Nevertheless, it's what you've got.

When you tell yourself, "I must be able to do what I want to do," but you can't because of circumstances beyond your control, then you feel sorry for yourself. Your mother's illness is such a circumstance. Accepting this reality, even when it's grim, helps you to develop more adaptive emotions and to cope better.

We can write a scenario for our future. It is totally appropriate to do so. It represents our hopes, our dreams, our aspirations, and it becomes our guide to actions that will help us to realize those hopes and dreams. We do our best to make this scenario come true. But if we say "It must come true," and obstacles occur, we become prisoners of our own insistent demands. Instead of disappointment, then we become angry or self-pitying—or both. It is certainly a great disappointment to see your hopes dashed.

Are you saying that it's appropriate to be disappointed?

Yes, of course. You raised your children, took care of your sick husband, and now you hope to do things for your own pleasure. And you can't, because of your mother's illness. Disappointment is an entirely understandable consequence. Your life has been drastically changed. And you are called upon to make new adjustments and new decisions daily—and sometimes from moment to moment. But how does it help you to add self-pity to your problems?

Let's look at the evening when your mother wandered away just when dinner was ready. Let's see what can be learned from that episode. Your mother wandered off when your back was turned. When you saw her down the street, you grabbed your coat and ran after her. Understandable. Your concern at the moment was for her safety. But you neglected to do one small thing before you started to look for her.

What was that?

Turn off the burner under the stew. If you had done that, your dinner would not have burned and been ruined. You would have calmed yourself down after you came back and served dinner to both of you.

Are you saying that it was my fault that dinner was ruined?

No, it wasn't your fault, or your mother's. Assigning blame solves nothing. Your mother wandered off because something in her disordered brain impelled her to do that. We don't know why AD patients wander, but they do. So it's wise to expect this and to secure the locks on doors to guard against that possibility. It's also wise to expect any unexpected or unexplainable behavior. That happens. Your mother's behavior does not and cannot respond to rational decision making and choices. But yours can. One of the most rational decisions you can make is to try to change your expectations of your mother.

What expectations? I no longer expect anything of her.

When you asked her to wait on the porch until dinner was ready, you expected that she would remember what you said. But she has a very short memory, a very poor sense of time, and occasional disorientation of place. If you really accept that, you will not expect normal behavior of her—even with respect to a simple request like "Wait here and I'll come for you when dinner is ready." You would not feel nearly so frustrated when she behaves in her own irrational manner.

How would that help me to stand this better?

When you expect normal behavior and are confronted with irrational behavior, you, too, become somewhat irrational and say to yourself, "This shouldn't be! I can't stand it!" But, tell me, why shouldn't she behave in this irrational, unpredictable manner?

I guess there's no reason why she shouldn't.

Then why does she?

Because her deteriorated brain guides her unpredictable behavior.

Yes, just as a normal brain guides normal behavior. And if you continue to keep that fact in the forefront of your thinking, you will be less likely to get as upset when she does unpredictable things. And you will be able to stand it better. When you stand it better, you'll be less likely to get stuck in self-pity.

We constantly alert ourselves to different expectations and different dangers in our environment. For example, when driving a car on a speedway, we are alert to one set of possibilities; when driving on a

crowded city street, to another; when caring for a
toddler, skiing down a slope or studying for a critical
exam—all gear us to different possibilities and prepare
us for different contingencies.

Over time, these expectations become automatic, and
we no longer consciously think of them. For example,
your first concerns the other day were your mother's
whereabouts and her safety. So you ran out to look
for her, but before you did, you automatically reached
for your coat because that is the result of a lifelong
habit. Looking around to see if any possible dangers
exist is not automatic now, but it is a new habit you
can learn.

Caring for a dementing loved one, because the sick
individual's behavior is not predictable, places an
enormous burden upon you. The responses that you
have learned throughout your lifetime often seem inadequate to the task. In fact, they often *are* inadequate. So you become frustrated and discouraged.

So what do I do now?

Practice new responses. Some of these will be practical, like eliminating environmental hazards that might
hurt your mother. Others will be behavioral, like learning to do old routines differently. Still others will be
cognitive, and these are primary.

I understand the practical and the behavioral, but give me an
example of the cognitive.

A new cognitive response would be saying to yourself, "She's doing what she's doing because that's what
her brain tells her to do. . . . She is not the same
person I once knew. She has lost the flexibility to

have options. But I haven't. I can choose not to upset myself unduly about what she does—even though I hate the position I'm in, and I still think it's unfair."

It is!

———•———

There seems to be no end to the changes I have to face. Every week, just as I get used to doing things I never had to do, or didn't think I would ever have to do, or didn't know how to do—new responsibilities crop up. Sometimes I feel that it's just too much for me.

In what way is it too much for you?

It's beyond my capacities. Sometimes I worry what will become of me and my wife if I give out. I feel very sorry for both of us.

Try to be specific. Tell us more about the changes you are going through.

Since my wife's illness has made it impossible for her to do the housework, I have had to take over. We have a housekeeper in once a week for a few hours. That's all I can afford. I do the rest. I never realized how much was involved—the shopping, the cooking, the laundry. We used to entertain. We used to go places. That's over.

My mother and my wife were both excellent cooks. So I guess I'm spoiled a bit. Now I do the cooking. I'm no gourmet chef, but I've learned to prepare steak-and-potatoes meals adequately. Before I leave for work, I prepare a sandwich for Jennie's lunch. Sometimes she doesn't remember to eat it.

I come home from work at about six, fix dinner, wash up, get Jennie ready for bed, watch the news on TV, and go to bed.

The next day is a repetition of the day before, except on some days Jennie seems worse than others. Those are the hardest. I don't know how much longer I can leave her alone.

On Saturdays, which used to be my health-club day, I take the laundry to the laundromat, do the marketing, and buy whatever the household needs.

On Sundays, I pay the bills, check over the accounts, and try to take Jennie for a little outing. Sometimes she gets so obnoxious that I have to turn around and come home, like last Sunday.

What happened last Sunday?

Last Sunday I decided that it would be nice if we went out to lunch. Just for a change of scene for both of us. So I took her to a local diner. Jennie read the menu for at least fifteen minutes before she decided on a sandwich. When it came, she insisted that that was not what she ordered. She wanted what I had. So we switched. She didn't like my sandwich and refused to eat. When the bill came, she asked to see it. She made a big scene, saying they were thieves, that they were overcharging, and that I shouldn't pay it. I calmed her down by assuring her that I would pay only a fraction of what they asked. That satisfied her. But I left the diner pretty shaken. And that ended my good intention of providing a pleasant outing on Sunday. That fiasco put me down in the dumps for the rest of the day. I don't know how long I can take this. I feel devastated.

What you're being asked to do is extremely difficult. Your wife's illness has enmeshed you in ways that you did not anticipate. It has changed not only her life, but yours also. You are constantly called upon to attend to the needs of another person. Your own needs get shunted aside. Your life has become constricted. To like this would be inhuman. To feel devastated only adds to your woes.

I do, indeed, feel devastated. How can I not feel devastated when I see my wife, with whom I have shared my life, deteriorate almost beyond recognition? How can I not feel devastated when I see my life, or what's left of it, slip away in an endless routine of pain and sorrow?

The pain and the sorrow are there. But the sense of devastation and the self-pity can be changed.

How?

Are you saying "This shouldn't, absolutely shouldn't, be happening to me"?

Yes, I think I am. Why should it be happening to me? I've never done anything to deserve this. Neither has Jennie. Why us?

One answer would be "Why not?" Tragedy is as much a part of life as triumph, sickness as much as health. People experience good outcomes and bad outcomes. Do you believe bad things happen only to people who deserve punishment?

No. I know that people don't always get what they merit, good or bad. I don't believe in perfect justice in the universe.

So, there is no reason why this should, or shouldn't, be happening to you. It just is. If you could change that fact, that would be great. But can you change it?

No.

Then by clinging to the "should not"—"This shouldn't be happening to me"—you are adding the burden of an irrational demand to the very real problems you already have.

What can I do?

You can change your thinking from "This shouldn't be happening to me" to the more realistic and rational "I wish this weren't happening. It's not what I want, but it's what I've got, and I'll try to make the best of it."

I agree with you. I know that what you say is true, and I accept it intellectually. But I don't feel it emotionally.

That's because you don't fully believe it. Your emotions respond to your beliefs, and your beliefs don't change overnight. Every time a difficult situation arises—as it will—you say something like "It's awful," and then you feel devastated. To change, it's necessary to do two things: first, give up the old belief that "It's awful," and second, practice the new belief that "It's sad but tolerable." And then it's necessary, just as with any new skill that you are learning, to practice, practice, practice, until the new response becomes automatic. Then you will feel less devastated.

I'll try to do that. But that's not all.

What else?

I know that Jennie is suffering. Sometimes she screams for no good reason—or none that I can figure out. Sometimes she just sits in a chair and seems out of it. And sometimes she says, "I want to die." And when that happens, I get a real pain in my stomach. I feel so deeply for her. And I feel so helpless.

You are, in fact, helpless to change her condition. You can only do what you can to make her more comfortable. But as for yourself, this is the time to start practicing what we call *emotional distancing.*

What is that?

It's a process of gradually withdrawing your emotional investment, built up over long years of marriage.

Are you suggesting that I stop caring about her altogether? Or become callous to her suffering.

Not at all. Emotional relationships aren't that black or white. In between the deep attachment you have developed and complete unconcern is a vast middle ground. What we are suggesting is a subtle process, which you probably have been experiencing to some extent without being aware of it. We think it is more adaptive to practice this on a more conscious level of awareness.

What do you mean?

During the course of a marriage, your lives become deeply intertwined. You become sensitized to each other's feelings, mood, pain, happiness. You may react positively or negatively to each other's feelings, states of mind, and well-being. But you generally react.

But now, your wife is changing. She is hardly the person you knew and with whom you built up a relationship over the years. She is no longer a person you can talk to, or with whom you can share any of your thoughts or feelings, pain or pleasure. So, in many fundamental ways, your relationship has changed. At the same time, you try to cling to the relationship that you have known. And that becomes more and more difficult, and eventually impossible. So, as part of you continues to care for her, and to love her for what she was—and still is—part of you removes yourself from the person she is becoming: dependent, demented, and unpredictable. You may continue to love her, and she may continue to love you.

But you can no longer expect your relationship to be reciprocal. Emotional distancing helps you to accept that. It's a process of emotional withdrawal.

Yes, I believe that some of that withdrawal has been happening. How can I do that on a conscious level?

You can say to yourself, "This is not the Jennie I once knew. She is deteriorating. I can continue to love her. And I do. I can only do my best for her. And I accept the fact that she can do little, if anything, for me. I feel for her pain and suffering, but I cannot immerse myself in it. Part of me had better remain apart from it. In that way, I can continue to do my best for her, and for me."

Sometimes I have said to myself, "I have lost my best friend." And that thought has been crushing. That's when I feel the worst.

Yes, indeed, you have lost your best friend. There is often a deep sense of loss when a spouse has AD. The outside—the appearance—seems intact, while the inside—the mind—crumbles. This feeling of grief is an appropriate emotional response to such a loss. But grief won't become devastation if you keep telling yourself, "I cannot be crushed by this. I am standing it."

———•—•———

We've been married for thirty-five years. We had our moments, our misunderstandings, our quarrels. But we both felt that we had a good relationship, that we understood each other and loved each other. Until about five years ago, when he began to change—subtly at first, so that you'd hardly notice anything different. Then it became apparent that something was wrong. When I realized that his mind was going and his personality was changing, I became frightened. My doctor sent us to a neurologist, then to a neuropsychologist, then to a special clinic for evaluation. The diagnosis was AD. I had never heard of this. Senility? Impossible. He was only sixty!

I covered for him a good deal. I helped him dress and bathe, and I took him for walks. I supplied the names he forgot, and the dates he confused, and the cues for time and place that he jumbled. I thought I had everything under control. I thought that if I were sensitive enough, and caring enough, and patient enough, that we could manage to weather this without too much difficulty.

Then what?

One day he screamed at me and accused me of stealing his hairbrush. He picked up the phone and tried to call the police. Fortunately, he didn't remember the number. At that point, I felt that I couldn't take any more. I felt that all the control I had built up was just like putting my finger in the dike.

What did you do?

At first, I couldn't believe that he meant it. So I asked him why I would want to steal his hairbrush. After all, I have my own. And I showed it to him. He didn't seem to hear me, or want to hear me. He looked at me menacingly and said to stop treating him as if he didn't know what he's talking about. He said that he put his brush down on the night table and it's not there now. So, obviously, I took it.

I patiently suggested that he might have put it somewhere else. At that, with a kind of wild look in his eyes, he said, "Are you telling me that I'm crazy?"

What went through your mind at that point?

I said to myself, "Yes, you're crazy! How much crazier are you going to get? How much craziness can I stand?"

How much craziness do you think you *can* stand?

I don't know. Sometimes I don't know who's crazier, he or I. Sometimes I feel that the world I knew is slipping from me. Sometimes I hate him, and sometimes I hate myself for hating him.

Yes, and if you acknowledge your true feelings, as you just did, you won't have to exercise as much control as you had been doing. Did you believe that as long as you were good, kind, patient, and understanding, that you would be repaid by "good" behavior and by gratitude, not by accusations of stealing his possessions?

Yes, I suppose I did.

And so you exercised what amounted to almost total control of your feelings to maintain that perfect image of the perfect wife, the perfect caregiver.

Well, what am I supposed to do, berate him for forgetting? Scream when he asks me the same question over and over again? Tell him "Yes, you're crazy," when he accuses me of stealing his hairbrush? Because that's what I really feel like doing.

That would only make matters worse. But, by recognizing, rather than denying, the emotions that his illness quite understandably arouses in you, you are in a better position to deal with them. You are right, the control you exercised was holding your finger in the dike to stem the tide. When the pressures build up, the flood waters break out and engulf you. But by recognizing that you can't always contain his outrageous behavior, that it will erupt in spite of your best efforts, you will not be so disturbed when he does outrageous things, such as accuse you of stealing his brush, or wallet, or shirt.

Then how shall I deal with my feelings?

First of all, by recognizing that it is normal and human to have them. Second, by recognizing that you have the human capacity to change the maladaptive feelings to more appropriate and adaptive ones.

First you tell me that it is normal and human to have feelings. And then you tell me to change them. How? By denying them? Or by yelling and screaming?

No. We are not suggesting that you deny your feelings, or suppress them, or give unrestrained expression to them. You can change your feelings by changing the way you interpret the events of your life.

How can I not feel hurt or sorry for myself when he makes those accusations against me? Those are my feelings. I have a right to them.

Yes, you do. And if you want to keep them, then you will, no matter what we say or do. But if you agree that hurt feelings and self-pity are neither necessary nor helpful for you, then you can change your emotions to sorrow or disappointment. You can do this by asking yourself, "How does a demented person act?" The answer is, of course, "Dementedly." If you give up all previously learned standards of behavior and substitute that simple statement, you will be able to tolerate his irrational behavior and irrational accusations more easily. And you will not attempt to reason with him, because you will know that he is unable to respond to reasonable arguments.

Then, you will be better prepared for the new surprises that will inevitably come. You will be able to withstand them better.

———•—•———

I never in my life held a hammer in my hand. I never had to. Paul was very good at those jobs around the house, and furthermore, he enjoyed doing them. Now I'm the fix-it man. Or is it fix-it woman? I grew up in an era when girls weren't even supposed to know one end of a nail from the other. Safety pins, yes, but nails and hammers, no. It wasn't "feminine." So now, at this point in my life, I have to change the broken doorknob, put a new valve on the hissing radiator, replace the broken slat in the venetian blind, change washers in the leaky faucet—all in addition to taking care of Paul—dressing him, bathing him, shaving him, and trying to keep him from blowing up or wandering away.

In addition, I have to pay the bills, balance the checkbook, and make all the decisions myself. I don't even have anyone to discuss things with. It's so hard.

Yes it is. But is "hard" the same as "impossible"?

No, it isn't.

And who said it should be easy?

No one. But why should this tragedy have befallen me?

Can you answer that yourself? Why you?

There is no reason. It just did.

Do you think that you were singled out for this painful situation by some special fate?

No, I don't think I was especially singled out. But it's terrible just the same.

Saying that it's terrible makes it much harder to bear.

Why?

Because words, like images, have great power to shape our emotions. When you use highly overcharged and loaded words like "terrible" or "awful" to label your situation, the emotions they evoke tend to be overcharged as well. You tend to see your situation in absolute, black-or-white terms, with no room for ameliorating circumstances or features. It's like saying "This is unbearable." But *is* it unbearable?

Yes, it is unbearable!

Aren't you bearing it?

Yes, I am.

Then it's difficult, but not unbearable. Every time you say to yourself, "This is terrible, this is unbearable," you add to the difficulty.

Are you saying that all I have to do is say the right words, and my problems will disappear? Like a magic incantation?

Not at all! There's no magic. If you give up calling it "terrible" and "unbearable," your problems will still be there. You won't feel great, but you won't feel awful, either.

I still don't understand. How will words change my feelings? They are only words.

Let's not underestimate the power of words. We use words to express our thoughts, but words serve a two-fold function. Not only do they mirror or reflect our beliefs, but they also shape and alter them. We can actually change beliefs and attitudes by changing the words we use. And since emotions follow logically from beliefs, we can change our feelings in this way as well.

Here's an example: Suppose you want to go to the beach, and you believe it would be terrible if rain prevented you from doing what you want. Then if it rains, you will probably say, "It's terrible that it is raining just when I wanted to go to the beach." And you will probably feel pretty miserable.

But suppose you say instead, "It's too bad that it's raining today; I'll have to change my plans and go to the beach another time." These words will shape a *new* belief, namely that the rain is unfortunate but hardly awful, and lead to a *new* feeling, namely disappointment. When you feel merely disappointed, rather than miserable, you can go about making other plans for the day.

By changing the words, you are actually re-educating yourself. We have been programmed to speak and think in hyperbole—in exaggerated and black-or-white terms. Things are "awful" or "terrible," "marvelous" or "dreadful." These terms leave no room for flexibility, for shades of gray, in thought and feelings. Changing the words to "sad" or "unfortunate" leads to internalization of a new set of beliefs, a set of beliefs that is more adaptive and offers greater behavioral choices.

I see that. But can changing words change the loneliness? Old friends have drifted away. I don't blame them. No one wants to put up with someone not in full possession of his faculties. People become embarrassed. They don't know how to react or what to say. And I have just stopped making the effort to maintain a social life.

Yes, unfortunately, it's true that people often drift

away. That's why women whose husbands have AD are often called "married widows." They find themselves in the anomalous position of neither having socially viable husbands or being free.

But why have you given up completely on having a social life? Are you perhaps contributing to your isolation in some way? Are you withdrawing from contacts?

Sometimes I feel ashamed of his behavior. I don't want to face anyone. It's too embarrassing.

Alzheimer's is a disease, not a disgrace. If you really believe that, you will stop feeling ashamed.

I know, but still I prefer not to impose this on anyone else.

What about your children?

My son lives on the other side of the country. He's very sympathetic, but there's nothing he can do. My daughter lives about an hour's drive from me. She's concerned; she calls about once a week to find out how we're doing. I always tell her we're doing just fine.

Why do you say that? Can't you be honest?

Margaret leads her own life. And it's a very busy one, with two young children and a career. I certainly can't expect her to do anything for me.

Why not?

Because I'm sure she must know how hard it is for me, and she has never volunteered to help.

Why do you have to wait for her to volunteer? Why can't you ask her?

Because I believe that my husband's care is my responsibility, not hers. I certainly don't want to be an overbearing or demanding mother who imposes her problems on her children.

Isn't there a distinction between an overbearing mother and one who reaches out to her daughter for help when she needs it? An overbearing mother is one who makes unnecessary and unreasonable demands in order to satisfy her own neurotic needs. We are not suggesting that you "impose" your problems upon your daughter. We are suggesting that her father's illness is her problem also. It's a family problem— your son's, too!

We suspect that at the same time that you tell your daughter "We're getting along just fine," you resent her for not knowing that you're *not* doing just fine. Is that true?

Yes, I suppose it is.

Then are you asking her to have ESP and to divine just how tough things really are? And do you really expect her to come running to help even though you assure her that you don't need help? Are you still playing the all-nurturant, protective mother to your "little girl" at the same time that you are the sole caregiver to your sick husband?

Maybe. I guess I've always been the one to take care of everyone.

Yes, that's what most women have been programmed to do, even at the expense of their own health and well-being. And they often feel that to ask for help demeans and belittles them in one of the few areas that allows them competence. You're always supposed to be the healer and the fixer, not of radiator valves but of people, especially of your own family.

Well, your daughter is a grown woman who doesn't have ESP, and she is probably willing to lend a hand now and then—if you discuss reality with her. Why don't you try it?

What shall I do? How shall I start?

Call her and tell her exactly what's going on. Tell her that from now on you are going to confide in her. Tell her how lonely you feel.

But I don't like to be a complainer.

There's a difference between being a complainer and being honest. Honesty about her father's condition and about your difficulties in dealing with it can only strengthen your relations with your daughter. And as her understanding increases, you can begin to ask her for some help. She will, in all likelihood, feel closer to you and to her father and to the whole process of his illness and the changes this has brought about in the family structure. You might even ask her to stay with her father now and then so that you can begin to go out and reconstruct your own social life.

That's not the same as being a complainer. A complainer whines for attention but shies away from problem solving. What we are suggesting *is* problem solving.

What if she refuses to do anything?

Are you afraid to ask her? Are you afraid that she will, in fact, refuse?

No, not really. But she might.

Let's assume that she does refuse. Would you take that as a rejection of you?

Perhaps I would feel that way.

Let's assume that you do ask her to help you and she refuses, either directly or by making lame excuses—or what you interpret as excuses. She may or may not have valid reasons. Where is the evidence that this would represent a rejection of you?

There is none.

Then let's separate the two possibilities. One is that her refusal is a rejection of you. The other is that she refuses because of reasons of her own. You admit that there is no evidence that the first is likely. Then any refusal on her part would probably relate to her own problems, such as the demands of her career or of her own family.

Yes, that's true.

Then what do you lose by speaking to her about it?

Nothing. In fact, I think she would probably do whatever is possible.

Fine. And you say you have no one to discuss anything with. How about your son? You say he's sympathetic, but he lives too far away to help. The phone crosses state and even national lines. How about talking things over with him, too?

Your son and your daughter are natural resources— probably your best. Why not start with them? And then we can discuss your joining a family support group for caregivers of AD patients.

Instead of Saying . . .	**Tell Yourself . . .**
I can't stand it!	I am standing it to the best of my ability.
Why did this happen to me?	There's no reason why this happened to me. It just did.
It's not fair!	The world is not fair. I'll do my best to accept what I can't change.
I am devastated.	I feel sad.
I don't deserve this.	AD is not a punishment inflicted upon me. I am doing my best in a difficult situation.
He shouldn't make ridiculous accusations against me.	Why shouldn't he make ridiculous accusations? It would be better if he didn't, but he is not able to make rational distinctions. However, I can!

CHAPTER 8

Guilt: I Should Have . . . I Shouldn't Have

Things have been going from bad to worse since Allen was diagnosed as having Alzheimer's disease last year. Naturally, many things have changed in our lives. We don't go out much. We don't see many people. There have been times when the going was pretty rough. But since last Monday, I've been feeling the lowest I've felt since Allen took sick.

What happened last Monday?

Last Monday night, I woke up at about 1 A.M. and saw that Allen was not in bed. I got up to look for him. He was wandering around in the living room in a dazed manner, muttering under his breath. I gently led him back to bed. He fell asleep.

About an hour later, I heard him get up again and make for the stairs to the basement. I jumped out of bed and again brought him back. I assumed he was settled in for the night. So I counted sheep, and in a little while I dozed off to catch what was left of the night.

Some time later, I heard banging on the piano. It was Allen. At that, I couldn't contain myself. I rushed into the living room. I asked what the hell he thought he was doing at that hour of the night.

Didn't he have any consideration for anyone? And I ordered him to go back to bed that very minute. I was beside myself. And then . . .

Go on, what happened?

I'm ashamed to tell you. I feel like a dog.

Say it. We can deal with it.

He flew into a rage, a terrible rage. He picked up an ashtray I had on a table and hurled it against the wall. He shouted obscenities. He threatened to leave and never come back. I was frightened. This was so unlike him. At first I thought of calling the police, but then I thought better of it. Eventually, he calmed down and went back to bed. But I was so ashamed of what I had done.

Ashamed of what you had done? What had you done?

I caused this wild episode.

How did you cause it?

By the way I reacted to his getting up during the night. I feel that I let him down by shouting at him so angrily when I found him at the piano. I could have found a better way of handling the situation.

Perhaps you could have found a better way. But are you saying that you should have?

Could have, should have—what's the difference?

The difference is vital to your emotional well-being. It is the difference between feeling regretful about the incident and feeling guilty. It is the difference between accepting your human fallibility and demanding perfection of yourself.

How?

"Should have" is an imperative. It is an absolute that expresses a command and doesn't allow for any exceptions, modifications, or limitations—no ifs, ands, or buts. No allowance for human limitations. It expresses the belief that you absolutely must have found a better way, and that if you didn't, you are lacking in some basic attribute of decency. The result of "should have," then, is self-downing and guilt.

"Could have" is a conditional statement that expresses a possibility. Perhaps you could have found a better way. Perhaps not. The fact remains that you didn't. Then why are you so blameworthy?

Because if I had not responded so heatedly, Allen would not have had that catastrophic reaction.

How do you know that?

I don't know it for sure, but it certainly seemed likely. It followed immediately after I blew up at him.

There's a common fallacy that if B follows A, then B is caused by A. If thunder follows lightning, can we say that it is caused by lightning? Obviously not. But perhaps they are both caused by a common set of circumstances—that is, atmospheric conditions.

Isn't it likely that your husband's outburst was caused by the same inner turmoil that motivated him to get up for the third time in one night? And that his rage was the culmination of the mental storm that was building up within him?

Yes, it's possible, but are you saying that my behavior had nothing to do with it?

No, we're not saying that. We don't know what triggers these emotional storms. It's possible that it could have been averted by some other behavior on your part. But there's no way we can be certain of that. We're dealing with a mind whose workings are unknown to us.

Are you saying that you should have known exactly what to do in a situation without precedent for you and under circumstances that are most trying and would be most trying for most people? And that if his response is frightening, uncontrollable, and outrageous, that it is all your fault?

I guess so.

Then perhaps you feel that you are called upon to be more than human.

What is more than human?

Perfect is more than human. Because humans are imperfect and live in an imperfect world. We are fallible creatures and prone to make mistakes. So if you truly believe that you must be infallible, you will put yourself down, heap blame upon yourself, and then feel guilty, when you perceive yourself to be less than perfect.

Guilt is the punishment you inflict upon yourself for the "crime" of having human limitations, for this is how you see it when you adopt such a perfectionist viewpoint. When you say to yourself that you "should" anticipate and fix Allen's moods, you are making demands upon yourself that deny your human limitations. Such demands are unrealistic. They assume that his behavior is under your control. Where is the evidence that this is possible?

Actually, there is none.

Then suppose you give up the idea that you have unlimited control over his behavior and your own responses.

Then are you saying that my angry response was justified because I'm human and fallible?

No, it's neither to be justified nor condemned. Angry responses do occur, and they can, to a considerable extent, be changed by using the methods we discussed earlier. What we are saying is that you can look at your own response and learn how not to become so enraged in the future. In that way, you recognize the inappropriateness of your response, without damning yourself as a guilty sinner, or a miserable person, for having reacted in the way that you did.

And how does one inappropriate response, in a very tough situation, make you a miserable person?

I guess it doesn't. But that's how I saw myself.

Yes, and that's why you felt so guilty. You judged yourself on the basis of one undesirable behavior. But one inappropriate response—or even several inappropriate responses—hardly add up to the sum total of who and what you are. Obviously, you are a person who behaves in many different ways, in different situations, and at different times.

You can change behaviors you don't approve of. When you separate the undesirable behaviors from the totality of you as a person, you will give up the self-punishment we call guilt. You will find the way to change the "should have" to "could have" and come up with better resolutions for future unexpected situations. And they won't be perfect.

I'll try, but it's difficult.

Yes, it's difficult—but it's more difficult *not* to. As Allen's condition worsens, it will get harder for you to anticipate his moods. His behavior will become more unpredictable. It will become increasingly important for you to be able to accept those things that are beyond your control—without blaming yourself. And to accept your own mistakes without condemning yourself as a rotten person for having made them.

How do I do this?

One way is to recognize the distinction between actions that are due to honest error or human failings and those that society views as crimes.

Errors are potentially correctible. They represent the *normal* course of human learning, adapting, and coping. Since nothing in your past experience has prepared you for the challenges of caregiving for an Alzheimer's victim, you will have to learn as you go. There is no way we know of for you to learn without errors. Crimes, on the other hand, are reprehensible behaviors that society agrees merit punishment. Doing less than you could, or having troubling thoughts, are not crimes.

You just mentioned troubling thoughts. I have some that trouble me a good deal. I have some pretty rotten thoughts. And I feel pretty rotten for having them.

Like what?

Sometimes I want to run away—a million miles away—and be free of it all. And then I feel awful for having such thoughts. And that's not the worst of it.

What's the worst?

Well, for example, the day after that big outburst, Allen was very quiet and subdued. I saw him sitting by the window, staring out. He looked so pathetic, even frightened. I couldn't help thinking of how he must be suffering. He was such a vital, strong, and creative man, and now he can't even dress himself, or figure out how to open a can. I almost wished for an end. You know, I began to have those terrible thoughts like . . .

Like what?

Like wishing he were dead. And then I hate myself.

Why do you hate yourself for having these thoughts?

Because first I tell myself that I wish it for his sake. That would end his suffering. And then I know that I'm wishing it for my sake, because that would end my tremendous burden of caring for him. And then I wish I were dead—that would put an end to the whole painful process of his slow death and my hopeless life. These are terrible thoughts, and I shouldn't have them.

Why not?

That's obvious. Because it's shameful. What kind of person would have such thoughts?

A person like you, or us, or any of the millions of caregivers in the United States today. That's who.

In the vicious cycle of anger, shame, and guilt, you have feelings or thoughts, such as wishing to be free, that you label as "bad" or "unacceptable" and then try to deny or repress. You do this because you mistakenly believe that to acknowledge them would make you a bad or unacceptable person. You don't distinguish between the *thought* and the *person* who thinks. Sometimes, no matter how hard you try to push them away, these thoughts and feelings occur anyway, because you are human, and it is human to get impatient, angry, or frustrated, to have less-than-admirable thoughts. Then you globally damn yourself as an awful person. And then you feel guilty.

Your thoughts of running away, your wish for Allen's death, or your own death, are not to be taken literally. They add up to a wish to be free of your burden. The wish to be free of this burden is understandable and well-nigh universal to caregivers. In fact, you would need the patience of a saint and the nobility of an angel in order *not* to have such thoughts from time to time. But you are neither saint nor angel, merely human, and therefore limited. So, you make mistakes, lose patience, get angry, and think thoughts of which you aren't proud. This is to be expected. You can learn to manage better and to moderate or alter such thoughts and feelings. But you can learn to accept them when they do occur.

What happens when you demand that you should not have such thoughts or feelings, when you tell yourself that you are a terrible person for having them?

I feel awful—guilty, ashamed, and inadequate.

Right! By demanding that you be more than human, you actually make yourself feel like something less.

So what do I do if I keep having these terrible thoughts?

Recognize that they are par for the course for caregivers. Expect that the wish to be free will recur, and don't condemn yourself when it does. Accept yourself even if you deplore the thoughts or feelings you may experience from time to time. Stop telling yourself you shouldn't or mustn't have them. For an imperfect human being, as we all are, this is like demanding that night not follow day. It simply isn't realistic.

Consider this: If you were on a jury trying a person for thoughts of running away, or wishing a sick, dependent person dead, or wishing one's self dead, would you condemn that person to prison?

No, of course not. They haven't done anything harmful.

Then why condemn yourself to the punishment of guilt for the same crime?

But don't you say that we feel and act how we think?

Yes, that's true. We do. But are you suggesting that these "reprehensible" thoughts are a prelude to reprehensible actions?

No, of course not.

Let's clarify some reasons why we agree with you that these negative thoughts are not instigators of reprehensible actions.

In the first place, your thoughts, in this case, represent wishes, not intents. And your wish is not to do harm to yourself, or your husband. Rather, as we said, you want to be free of a great and painful burden. That's understandable. And, as the old saying goes, "If wishes were horses, beggars would ride."

In the second place, at the same time that you have these "reprehensible" thoughts, powerful inhibitors come into play. These inhibitors are your value system, built up over a lifetime. This value system says, "In spite of all the pain that he and I are experiencing now, I really don't want to desert him. I want to make life as bearable as I can for him." These are the thoughts that you accept as primary, because they are consonant with your value system.

These are what we call your *ego-syntonic* thoughts. They square with your values and with your sense of yourself as a responsible and decent person. "Chucking it all," while understandable, is *ego-dystonic*. That is, it violates your sense of yourself. So you reject it. The *ego-syntonic* thoughts are the ones that you act on.

Yes, that's true. That rings a bell. I really don't want to run away, and I really don't want either Allen or me to die. But sometimes I feel torn apart.

In what way?

I feel torn between wanting to do my best for him—what you call my *ego-syntonic* thoughts, and wanting to chuck it all—my ego-dystonic thoughts. Then I get a splitting headache.

Very understandable. Your inability to resolve the conflict between your desire to lead a more normal life, and your commitment to your husband, your value system, creates considerable stress, which expresses itself as a headache. This conflict results in what we call ambivalence—a yes-no situation.

Yes, I often do experience that kind of conflict. What can I do about it?

Acknowledge it. And accept it. Unfortunately, we live in a world that sends powerful messages to us, messages that state that there is a solution for every problem. Possibly a pill. Or if no pill is available, all conflicts can be resolved in a half hour, with three interruptions for station breaks and commercials. If we buy this message—and most of us do—then we feel powerless and guilty if we can't live up to it. We feel that we should not have conflicts, should not have to live with them, should be able to resolve them, and that if we feel ambivalent in a difficult situation, it's all our fault.

It isn't your fault, or your husband's fault. So accept the ambivalence as a natural part of the human condition, and don't add guilt to your burden.

———•·•———

Last month, I finally went away for a weekend—Saturday morning to Sunday evening. A friend of mine invited me to her house in the country and persuaded me to go. I called a home health-care agency and they sent me a lovely woman who seemed very experienced and competent. So I went.

I couldn't enjoy myself. I kept imagining that this woman wouldn't be nice to Richard, that he might become abusive to her, or that she might become abusive to him. I kept calling home to make sure that things were going right.

Then, when I came home, Richard looked at me as if I were a stranger. At first, he refused to talk to me. Then he broke down and cried.

You can imagine how I felt.

How did you feel?

Like a worm.

I see that we're back in the guilt trap. Why did you feel like a worm?

Because I saw how much it meant to him to have me home. It was as if I had abandoned him.

Do you feel that you abandoned him?

In a way, yes, I did abandon him. Because his need for me was greater than my need to take a weekend off.

How can you measure the one against the other? Is there a score sheet, a ledger, or a set of scales that gives you a definitive answer?

No. Not really.

Then how can you determine, at any one time, whose need is greater? And why measure yours against his? This puts a great deal of stress upon you. Do you feel that you must put aside all thoughts of your own well-being in order to be a good wife to your sick husband?

Perhaps not all, but I certainly should avoid doing anything that would hurt him. He's so totally dependent.

Yes, he is totally dependent. But is he totally dependent upon *you?* Was he well cared for in your absence?

Yes, physically he was well cared for. But emotionally, I could see that he was hurt by my absence.

Did his condition worsen because you were away for two days?

No.

Then why do you say that he was hurt by it? He obviously regained his fragile emotional equilibrium quickly enough on your return.

Do you feel that it's possible for you to provide him with a perfect world? That you can cushion him against all emotional pain?

Not all, but as much as possible.

How much is that?

I don't know.

Are you, perhaps, setting up some unrealistic standard of behavior for yourself? One that says that if he is emotionally pained because you have taken two days off for yourself, then you must feel guilty, and vow never, ever to do such a thing again? Aren't you being unduly self-punitive? Because guilt is an emotion that says, "I have done wrong, and I must be punished for it."

But isn't it selfish for me to think of myself? After all, he is the sick one. And he is suffering.

Don't forget that you are not dealing with an acute illness, where your intense and total devotion, for a limited time, may mean the difference between life and death. You are dealing with a chronic disease whose course is long and painful and whose end is certain. You are a party to this disease. Your life is intimately affected by it. It places serious constraints upon you.

That being the case, why is it selfish to allow personal considerations to enter into the overall picture of how best to deal with this illness? If you don't allow your own needs to weigh in your plans, then you will feel guilty, no matter how much time you devote to your husband. You will be aiming for a perfect solution for him, where no perfect solution is possible. You will feel that you failed him. There will always be things undone, needs unmet, critical situations unforeseen. Will you always heap "should haves" and "shouldn't haves" upon yourself to make you feel guilty?

Guilt can become an albatross upon your back, preventing you from making more appropriate decisions in a very difficult situation.

Do you think that you deserve the punishment of guilt because you took a two-day vacation?

Not if you put it that way. I never saw guilt as a punishment. I just saw it as a natural reaction. Something I feel. And that it's normal to feel that way. Especially if you have decent standards of behavior.

There's a difference between a decent standard of behavior and a self-image of perfection, selflessness, and nobility.

A decent standard of behavior involves caring, sharing, and giving. At the same time, it involves a recognition of the limits of what you can do for another person. Sometimes—as in the case of taking care of an Alzheimer's victim—it means stretching yourself beyond what you formerly thought were reasonable limits. But it doesn't mean stretching yourself to the breaking point. It doesn't mean total self-sacrifice. It doesn't mean martyrdom.

You have to decide for yourself what those limits are. Limits vary with different people: their personalities, their emotional makeup, their physical well-being, and their social and financial resources. But we all have limits. A recognition of these limits includes giving yourself permission to consider yourself as part of the family dyad—the sick member and the caregiver. Consideration for yourself may mean going out with friends once in a while, going to a movie or the hairdresser, or going away for a few days—whatever will give you some pleasure. And feeling secure in the knowledge that you are not hurting your loved one and that you deserve some pleasure.

If, on the other hand, you have a self-image of perfection and nobility, you will translate that into total selflessness. And, since total selflessness is an unrealistic ideal, you pay a price for trying to achieve and maintain that image. The price you pay is emotional upset. This is often in the form of anger with the sick person for constantly putting you in a position that tests your patience, forebearance, and noble intentions; frustration at your inability to foresee and control events; and guilt because you feel that it's all your fault.

Yes, but if you really cared for that person, wouldn't you want to put aside all personal consideration?

You are confusing caring for a person and caregiving. Caring for a person means love, concern, and commitment. Caregiving means taking care of that person. You can love your husband, show him all of the affection that you have, and at the same time share the caregiving with another person, be it a friend, a family member, or a paid helper. Doing so doesn't diminish your affection. And it doesn't tell you, or the world, that you are an uncaring person.

Then how can I do that without feeling guilty?

Tell yourself that guilt is a self-inflicted punishment for a perception of wrongdoing. Tell yourself that since you have done no wrong by doing something for yourself, and have hurt no one, you don't deserve punishment. Give yourself permission to take time off for yourself.

And change the "should haves" to "could haves."

Then examine your "could haves" and make rational guilt-free decisions for the future.

In your case, this translates into, "I could have stayed home for the weekend, but I chose not to." This eliminates guilt and opens the way to decide whether or not you would benefit from time off again.

———•———

I've been taking care of my wife ever since she came down with Alzheimer's disease a couple of years ago. It's been tough, but we manage to get by. I especially miss the chance to get together with some of my old pals from the plant. I'm retired and with Alma's illness, well, it's kind of hard to socialize. That's why I was so happy about going into town for an old friend's retirement dinner.

I arranged for my niece to come over and stay with Alma until I came home. I had to leave before my niece could get there, but I left a key for her with my neighbor. Shortly after dinner started, I got a call from my niece. When she arrived at my house, about an hour after I left, she found the door wide open, and Alma was nowhere to be found. She was frantic. I rushed home. We searched the neighborhood and finally called the police.

Alma was finally found, wandering around, confused, disoriented, and disheveled. I was devastated. I should never have gone to that dinner. I should have known better than to have left her alone, even for that short period of time. I never thought that she could unlock the door and let herself out. From now on, I'll never let her out of my sight.

With hindsight, it's clear that the preparations you made for your wife's supervision in your absence were inadequate. But you didn't have the benefit of hindsight when you made your plans for your evening out, did you?

No, but I should have foreseen the possibility.

How so?

Common sense tells me I should have, that's all.

While it's wise to expect the unexpected when dealing with a patient with a dementing illness, short of having a crystal ball, it's difficult to see how you could have predicted the exact events that did occur. But even if one argues that better plans *could* have been made—and in this case there are some practical steps to minimize the likelihood of a recurrence—does it follow logically that you absolutely should, *must* have done things differently?

Logically, no. But emotionally—here in my gut—yes.

Your emotional reaction—your gut feeling—stems from what's in your head. There is a logic to feelings, and as long as your head tells you that you should have foreseen the future and prevented it from happening, then you will feel overwhelming guilt.

What else can my head possibly tell me? I mean, look at what happened.

The outcome was unpleasant and frightening, but fortunately not disastrous. Even if it had turned out worse, it would not be necessary, or helpful, to blame and damn yourself for it. Nor would it be adaptive for you to withdraw and constrict your activities as a solution. No matter how diligently and conscientiously you devote yourself to your wife's care, your human limitations dictate that you will err and that you will fail to prevent unpleasant events from time to time.

So what do I do—tell myself that it doesn't matter?

No, because it *does* matter. One thing you are telling yourself that makes good sense is: "I wish I had planned more carefully for unexpected contingencies, and I will try to do better next time". Such self-talk generates appropriate and better adaptive emotions, like sorrow, regret, or disappointment, as well as motivation for future efforts. But it does not generate the guilt you felt. Guilt, which is dysfunctional, comes only if you add the maladaptive statements that "I must always prevent unpleasant outcomes" and "I'm a rotten person who deserves condemnation if I fail to do so."

You say that guilt is dysfunctional. I understand that means it doesn't help me to cope better with my situation. But isn't guilt sometimes beneficial? I mean, isn't that what prods us to mend our ways?

Many people believe this is true, but in fact the evidence is to the contrary. Because guilt involves self-downing and self-condemnation, it is more likely to lead to a self-fulfilling prophecy: "I am a rotten, worthless person who cannot possibly do anything right." Such thinking reflects a fairly common cognitive error, called *overgeneralization,* in which you fail to distinguish between an inadequate or careless act and the totality of the actor, or self. "I failed to do this well" is *not* the same as "I am a failure." For the same reason, perfectionism is less likely to motivate us to perform better than it is to create levels of anxiety high enough to interfere with performance. In your case, your guilt prompts you to withdraw and avoid, not to try again.

So what *does* keep us on track?

Concern for the patient, enlightened self-interest, and our own value systems. Since you genuinely care for your wife, her welfare is important to you, and you will tend to put forth the most effort on those areas of your life you find most significant. This is part of your value system. So is the responsibility you feel toward a helpless, dependent individual. It isn't necessary to beat yourself up in order to discharge the role you have voluntarily accepted. In addition, your own best interest is served by doing the best you can for your wife. When she is relatively comfortable, you can take time to attend to yourself. Ultimately, this is good for both of you.

You know, I've always thought that you *should* feel guilty when you do something wrong, that it's part of the process of atonement.

Atonement is defined as making amends for an offense or crime. For example, if you carelessly throw a ball through your neighbor's window while playing with your grandchild, you can make amends by replacing the window. There is no way you can undo what is done. Tell us, how does feeling guilty make amends for a negligent act?

Only symbolically, I guess—kind of like sackcloth and ashes. At least it shows how sorry I feel.

Do you think that symbols and abstractions have any meaning for Alma?

No, not anymore.

So whom are you trying to convince?

Myself, I suppose.

Why do you need convincing? You know very well how much you regret what happened. Perhaps you believe that doing something negligently or carelessly may not necessarily make you a rotten person—provided you conspicuously display the trappings of guilt, your sackcloth and ashes. Perhaps you believe that only by punishing yourself in this way can you prove your worthiness as a person.

So the guilt and the noble resolutions of self-sacrifice are just part of a superstitious ritual I'm going through to excuse myself?

Yes. Why not excuse yourself—which means accepting, rather than condemning, yourself for your human limitations—without the unnecessary added burden of guilt?

Is it realistic for you to promise yourself that you will never let her out of your sight again? Can you keep your eyes on her twenty-four hours a day, 365 days a year? Is it in your own long-term interest, or hers, to withdraw from social contact in this way and isolate yourself with only Alma for company?

No. But how else do I avoid making the same mistake again? This could easily have been a disaster. Who knows what might have happened to her? I feel so awful this time, I know I couldn't stand it if she came to some harm because of my negligence.

When you get a better handle on your own emotional reactions, you can then turn your attention to practical solutions. For example, how about getting your wife a nonremovable ID or MedicAlert bracelet so she can be brought home more easily if by any chance she does wander off? And next time, you can wait until your respite caregiver arrives before you leave for your appointment.

My parents are both in their late seventies. They have their own apartment not too far from mine. I'm the only daughter, and I have a younger brother. Dad is basically O.K. mentally—a little forgetful, you know—but physically, he's quite frail and not up to the daily chores like shopping, cooking, and cleaning. So I arranged for a homemaker and health aide, but my mother, who has Alzheimer's, is constantly finding fault and throwing them out for one reason or another— or for no reason at all. It seems like I'm the only one who can do anything for her, like she only wants me. Sometimes she even calls me in the middle of the night. Whatever time it is, I have to drop everything and go running. It's true I have no babies to take care of anymore—two of my children are on their own—but I do have a husband and a teenager at home, and they expect me to be there for them also. I feel like I'm at my wit's end, but I see no way out. My life is one mass of conflicting demands and I don't know what to do first. I'm constantly torn between my parents' needs and those of my own family.

So what do you do?

I tear my hair out and feel rotten no matter what I do. My daughter blasts rock music until all hours of the night, so I yell at her a lot, and I don't feel very good about that. I feel guilty about not giving her the time that a teenager needs. I was always there for the two older children during their teen years. I know she'd like me to be around to talk to, and to help her to plan parties for her friends— not to go running to Grandma's all the time. But I can't do all they expect of me.

Yesterday, my husband's boss gave a dinner party and we were expected to attend. Then Mom called and insisted I come right over. My husband was furious. He said, "You have obligations to us, too." Well, I didn't know what to do. I felt so overwhelmed, I just sat down and cried.

Feelings like "overwhelmed," "upset," and "miserable" often include a large measure of self-pity and guilt. Were you saying to yourself "Poor me. I should

be a good wife, a good mother, and a good daughter,
at all times"?

Probably. It's true. But, it seems that no matter how hard I try,
somebody isn't satisfied.

In this situation you cannot satisfy everybody because each has different and conflicting expectations
of you. This follows from the different roles you are
simultaneously playing: daughter and caregiver, wife
and mother. What has been lost in this welter of
conflicting demands is *you:* your own expectations of
yourself and your own life. Aren't you demanding
that you must do it all?

Well, who else is there? I mean, if I don't take care of my parents'
needs, nobody else will.

We aren't suggesting that you neglect your parents
or that you ignore their legitimate requirements. But
does that mean you must do everything your mother
wants whenever she wants it—"drop everything and
run," as you put it?

What choice do I have? Just last week she called at night, hysterical.
She'd fired the aide again. I had to go. I couldn't leave them alone.

There are two separate issues here. One is whether
you must, or even can, do everything your parents
want. The second is whether they can realistically
continue to stay in their own apartment if this is what
it takes for you to keep them there. Let's tackle these
issues one at a time.

Why must you do it all? What would happen if your
mother called and you weren't home, if you had taken
a weekend for yourself?

I don't know. I can't imagine doing anything like that.

Why not?

I wouldn't be able to relax. I'd worry about what was happening to them, and then I would feel guilty for not being there. It's easier if I stay close so I can smooth things over.

Smoothing things over is something you are probably very good at. After all, you have been practicing it, as a nurturer, for many years. But your mother's illness is a new challenge, something you haven't faced before, and it will take new responses on your part— and the rest of your family—to cope with it. If you jump out of bed at night to avoid worry or to avoid dealing with your feelings of guilt, then you are not facing the reality of your mother's illness. This does not make things easier in the long run. Look at how torn and conflicted you are feeling. Look at the difficulties that your running whenever Mom calls has caused in your own household. Consider the consequences to your own health of continued stress and loss of sleep. Is it really easier?

No, I suppose not. But what am I supposed to do?

Face the fact that you need not and cannot continue to do everything your parents want. Change what you are telling yourself about your responsibilities to them. Instead of saying, "I must go whenever Mom calls," tell yourself, "I do the best I can, but I don't have to do everything. Things don't have to be perfect for them."

O.K. So I can say that, but what if Mom gets so upset that she injures herself or destroys things? Or hurts Dad? She gets out of control at times. And when she is at her worst, that's when she fires her home health aide and insists that I come over.

If that's what's happening, then it may no longer be realistic for them to live alone. It sounds like this is the time for you to be looking into other alternatives.

Like what?

Like placement in a nursing home.

I can't do that.

Why not?

For one thing, about ten years ago, when Mom was just beginning to face old age—and fear it—she made me promise that, come what may, I'll never send her, or Dad, to a nursing home. And I promised. So, you see, I can't go back on my word.

Of course, when we give our word, we intend to keep it. But it isn't engraved in stone. There are extenuating circumstances.

I don't see how there can be. A promise is a promise.

Suppose you had promised your son that when he got his degree in business administration, you would set him up in a business of his own. And then suppose that subsequently you and your husband lost all your money through a series of reverses. Would you then still feel that you were honor bound to keep your promise?

No. Not if I didn't have the money.

What would you do?

I would explain the situation and hope that he would understand.

And if he didn't understand? And was angry? Would you feel obligated to give him money you didn't have?

No. I just would have to break my promise. And he would have to accept that.

O.K. Now let's look at your situation with your mother. Ten years ago, when both you and your parents were ten years younger and richer in energy, you made a promise never to send them to a nursing home. In other words, you promised to invest your future energies in their care. Now, ten years later, their needs are too great for your present level of energy and your immediate family's welfare. Then why is it wrong, under these changed circumstances, to go back on your word?

My parents would be very upset. Even my husband and daughter— although they resent the amount of time I spend at my parent's house— would condemn me for doing this. They know about my promise and believe that a promise is a sacred trust.

If a flood or earthquake destroyed your home, or injured one of your loved ones, or if you fell seriously ill, would you expect that life would go on exactly as before?

No, of course not. That would be impossible.

Well, what has happened to your parents is very much like that sort of catastrophic event, and it requires similar strategies in order to cope.

I know that my mother wouldn't understand. But my husband and daughter—what can I do about them?

How about sitting down and having a talk with them? Explain to them the impossible situation that you're in, what with their demands upon you, and your mother's demands. They may not even realize how this is affecting you.

But I would still feel guilty about putting such a burden on the rest of my family. This is really something for me to handle.

Members of the so-called "middle generation" such as yourself have many roles to play—independent adult, wife, mother, daughter, perhaps a career, too. One of the most basic roles you, as a woman, have been trained to fulfill is that of nurturer and caregiver, fixer of people's problems. These responses are, by now, so overlearned and automatic that it is difficult for you to step back and see that you are entitled to nurture yourself also. We have referred to the conflicting expectations that your husband, daughter, parents, and others have of you, and how impossible it is for you to satisfy all of them simultaneously. When you stop demanding of yourself that you must meet all their expectations and have their approval, you free yourself from the insoluble conflicts. You can then set limits, ask for help, refuse requests, take time for yourself—and do all these things without guilt.

You're right. I am very much in the middle. You know, my brother lives fairly close by, but he doesn't seem too interested in what's going on. He calls occasionally; he drops by once in a while; but he doesn't get involved. He seems to feel that this is my responsibility, not his.

Like so many women, you were raised to be all-giving and all-nurturing, in contrast to your brother, who internalized other messages and different priorities. However, it's not too late to involve him.

How?

Why not sit down with your husband, daughter, and brother, and talk it out? Family meetings are useful forums for making and modifying plans and for dealing with caregiving issues as they come up. We'll talk about family meetings in more detail later in the book.

———•—•———

Miriam has been sick for many years. And the last year has been most difficult. She's only occasionally aware of her surroundings. She remembers very little of what is said to her. She used to be a very verbal person, but now she garbles words and sentences. Sometimes I feel that I should send her to a nursing home. And then I reject the idea as unthinkable.

Why?

Because it doesn't seem right.

What's not right about it?

She's always loved her home. Did everything to make it attractive. I feel that I owe it to her to let her live out her life here. But there are other problems . . .

What are they?

She's become incontinent. I have a home health aide who comes in during my working hours. But I'm finding it harder and harder to cope with her care the rest of the time. I don't know what to do.

Many people find that when the Alzheimer's victim becomes incontinent, that is often the cue for nursing home placement. What is your objection to it?

For one thing, I've often thought that nursing homes are warehouses for the unloved and unwanted. Way stations on the road to death.

Some, unfortunately, are just that. But not all. If you shop around carefully, you will find that some are well run and attuned to the needs of the residents. Yet nursing-home placement is one of the most difficult decisions that many people face. And it is one of the most guilt-producing. Assuming that you can find a good one, what are some of your objections?

Every time I come close to making a decision to send Miriam to a home, I get pounced on from all sides. My sister-in-law calls me and says, "How can you do such a thing? Don't you care what happens to her?" And my son—who lives 1,000 miles away—says, "But she's my mother. I can't sleep nights thinking of her among strangers who won't give a damn about her." And then, when I think, "They're right, of course. How can I do such a thing?" my friend Jim, who sent his wife to a nursing home after her stroke, says, "Are you trying to be a martyr?" So, you see, I get hung somewhere in the middle.

The middle is an uncomfortable place to be. Are you there because you're trying to please everybody? Are you primarily concerned with what's best for Miriam and you? Or are you primarily concerned with what the others will think of you?

I want to do what's right.

Is there an absolute right or wrong decision? And if so, how will you arrive at it? Will you poll all of your friends and relatives? And since they will not all agree, will you let majority rule?

No, of course not.

Then let us suggest that this is a decision for you to make, based on Miriam's needs, your ability to satisfy them—either at home or in a nursing home— and your own needs. Leaving other people's opinions aside, at the moment, what do you think is the best solution?

I think she might be better off in a nursing home, if I can find a good one. But then I begin to feel very guilty.

Because?

Because I'm not sure whether I'm doing this for her sake or mine.

Let's assume that your interests are also part of the decision-making process. What's wrong with that?

I should be able to put my own interests aside.

Where is that written?

No place.

Then suppose you start by giving up the "shoulds." That's where your guilt is coming from. There are no "shoulds"—only choices. If you give up the "shoulds," you will be in a better position to make rational choices. Not perfect ones, since there are no perfect choices, but ones better attuned to the reality of the situation.

Well, suppose that I give up the "shoulds" and decide to send Miriam away. And I tell myself that I have no reason to feel guilty about that. And that I have no reason to feel guilty even if part of my decision is that it would also be best for me, because I really don't want to be a martyr. And then along will come my sister-in-law and make me feel like Jack the Ripper.

How can she make you feel like Jack the Ripper?

By telling me what an awful person I am for doing this to her sister.

You can't control what your sister-in-law says. But you can control your own response to it.

How?

By telling yourself, "That's her opinion. She's entitled to it. But I don't have to buy it." And say it over and over again until you really believe it. That goes for everyone else who disagrees with your decision, including your son, who loves his mother but is not responsible for her care.

Could anyone make you feel guilty if you didn't agree with what they were saying—that you were a terrible person for doing what you decided to do?

You mean, it's only if I say those same things about myself that I feel guilty?

Precisely.

O.K. So I don't condemn myself for my decision—and anyone who doesn't like it will have to come to terms with their own feelings. Right?

Yes. And remember in many respects, this is the ultimate question for all AD caregivers. The decision that one's own emotional resources have been exhausted and that the disease has progressed beyond the point of home care is probably the hardest one to make. To accept that the time has come to place one's mate in a nursing home is to acknowledge the grim reality of AD.

On the other hand, nursing-home placement is often in the best interest of the patient. It can provide a good, safe environment where the resident can meet other people his own age and participate in activities, however limited, geared to his abilities.

But I've heard that some people don't live very long after going into nursing homes; that seems like such a betrayal, like I'm sentencing her to death. How can I not feel guilty over that?

If that's how you view it, you will feel guilty. It is true that the move to a nursing home is sometimes followed by a swift, downward course. That is due partly to the stress of change, and also to the fact that caregivers tend to keep their relatives at home as long as possible, so the patient's condition is typically quite poor by the time the move occurs. But is it *you* who has written the death sentence, or is it the disease process itself?

Obviously, the disease. It's so unfair.

Yes, it is. But since you didn't ask for it, or do anything to bring it on, why not refuse to blame yourself for what you cannot control and not make yourself feel guilty about it?

———•———

I'm a high school teacher of English. I love what I do. I worked hard to get where I am. And now I'm faced with a terrible dilemma. My husband has AD. He can no longer be left alone. He needs help dressing and toileting. He wanders. He doesn't remember to eat lunch, even when I prepare it for him.

I look at my choices, and all seem wrong.

What choices do you see?

The first and most obvious would be to get a home health aide. That would enable me to continue to do what I do best—teach English in high school.

That sounds fine. What's wrong with that?

I've heard that good aides are few and far between. There aren't many who would have the qualities that I feel are necessary: understanding, patience, compassion. I would always be haunted by visions of Steve being abused, or neglected, or hurt.

Also, even if I found the right person, Steve seems to need me so much. When I come home from school, he gets very clingy, follows me around the house, like he's afraid of losing me. I even have trouble keeping him out of the bathroom when I use it. So how can I leave him with a clear conscience to another person?

Then there's a nursing home. I don't object on principle. I know that there are some good ones. But Steve doesn't seem to be a likely candidate for one—yet.

He has forgotten many people and places, but he has not forgotten his home, or me. He is still aware of what he built—the porch he added on with his own hands, the flower beds he dug and planted. He still enjoys our meals together, our little walks, sitting in the garden. I think that sending him away would be cruel and would hasten his deterioration.

That leaves me the third alternative.

Which is?

To quit my job and stay home with him. That's what my relatives, and his, think I should do. But that would drive me crazy.

Why?

I tell myself that that's what a good wife would do for the husband she loves. Well, I love him. But does that mean that I have to give up everything I strove for in order to take care of him?

It's not in my temperament to stay home and be the full-time devoted caregiver. I feel that I would shrivel intellectually. Especially devoting myself to a person who no longer responds to much. Does that make me out to be an ogre?

Suppose, for a moment, that you were a man. Do you think that a man would feel like an ogre if he didn't give up his career to take care of a sick wife?

No, he wouldn't. But I'm not a man.

We are not suggesting that you try to act like a man. We are suggesting that, as a full human being, you have the right of choice. And that continuing your career is a viable choice.

But part of me wants to stay home and take care of my husband.

Which part of you is stronger? The part that wants to stay home and be a full-time caregiver, or the part that wants to continue your career? Suppose you assign a percentage to each choice.

The part of me that knows that staying at home is something I was not cut out to do—that gets 80 percent.

That gives you your answer, doesn't it?

Yes, it does.

Then examine the two alternatives that you mentioned before. Between nursing home placement, and home health care, which do you think is preferable now?

Home health care.

Then suppose you do that. Without guilt. In spite of what anyone says. And remember, there are no perfect solutions. If Steve clings to you even more when you come home, that's just one more difficult behavior you will have to deal with.

The most difficult part—and the one only you are capable of solving—is to convince yourself that you are entitled to continue your career, while assuring good care for your husband.

Instead of Saying . . .	**Tell Yourself . . .**
I should have done better.	I did the best I could under the circumstances. I'll try to do better if I can.
I should be a perfect caregiver.	I'm a human being with limitations and flaws. Nobody's perfect.
I'm a rotten person for acting inappropriately.	I am not the same as my act. If my act was a poor one, that doesn't make me a rotten person.
I'm an awful person for thinking unacceptable thoughts.	Thoughts are not deeds. Having thoughts that I deplore simply means I'm human.
I should never get angry with my AD relative.	I can work to minimize my angry responses, but I'll try to accept myself if I do lose my temper from time to time.

Instead of Saying . . .	**Tell Yourself . . .**
I should be able to find a good solution to all problems.	Some problems don't have good solutions. Where is it written that they must, or that I must be able to find them?
I should put aside all my own needs to attend exclusively to my relative.	I do not have to sacrifice myself as a noble martyr in order to provide for my relative's care. Which is my goal—caring for my relative, or earning my halo?
I should feel guilty when I make mistakes or behave less than nobly. Guilt is a form of atonement.	Mistakes are neither sins nor crimes, but rather a normal part of human learning. Guilt does not undo or make amends for errors, so it is a waste of emotional resources.

CHAPTER 9

Anxiety: I Feel Threatened

It's been increasingly clear to me over the last few months that something is wrong with my husband, Lou, although I still don't know what it is for sure. We've been to a couple of doctors, and one of them referred us to a neurologist, who said it might be Alzheimer's. I don't even know what that means, but he said not to worry, he's still evaluating Lou. But how can I not worry? I feel like my whole world has been turned upside down. I can't eat, I have terrible dreams, and I feel impatient, tense, and edgy all the time. I am worried about Lou, about what is happening to him, what's going to happen, and what it all means.

Tell us what you see in your husband's behavior that leads to the conclusion that something is wrong.

Well, it doesn't happen all the time, but he sometimes doesn't seem to know where he is, or who I am, or what he has just been doing. He'll ask the same question over and over again, and doesn't seem to remember that he asked before—or that I answered. The first time that happened, I thought he was kidding. I got annoyed and let him know I didn't appreciate the joke. The hurt, confused expression on his face told me he wasn't joking. Well, that scared me.

What did you do?

I tried to forget about it. It didn't happen again, and for the next few days, he was his usual self. But then, as I was driving him home from the train one day, he looked at me so strangely and asked, "Where do I live?" I said, "You live at home with me and the children." Then he asked—and he was dead serious—"Who are you?"

How did you feel?

I panicked. I was petrified. I stopped the car, thank God, or I think I would have crashed it. My heart was racing, I felt like I couldn't breathe, and I couldn't stop shaking. At one point, I remember thinking I would pass out. Somehow, I pulled myself together and got home. I was so drenched with perspiration that I went right upstairs to shower and change. When I came down, Lou was sitting in his easy chair, reading the paper just as he always does. I asked him if he felt better. My voice was trembling, and I looked white as a sheet. Lou said he was fine, but I didn't look so good. It was obvious to me that he didn't remember the incident. But I can't forget it. And there have been others—like forgetting the names of our kids. I haven't had a peaceful night's sleep since. I keep wondering, what next?

What do you think will happen next?

I don't know. I think it's the uncertainty that's keeping me on edge. Even when Lou acts all right, I keep imagining awful things. Sometimes I feel my heart racing and that terrible choking sensation I had in the car, and I wonder whether I'm having a heart attack—or maybe losing my mind. I don't understand any of what's going on, and I can't take it much longer.

Do you have any reason to suspect you may have heart trouble?

No. In fact, when I first took Lou to the doctor, I used the excuse that we both needed checkups. He didn't want to go. I got a clean bill of health.

The symptoms you describe are not those of heart disease or mental illness, but rather those of an anxiety attack. The feelings are very unpleasant but not dangerous, and they pass. Such symptoms are generally triggered in situations in which we perceive threat or danger that we don't feel able to handle.

Well, that definitely describes my situation. I don't even understand it, let alone handle it.

Let's help you first to understand your own reactions when you experience anxiety symptoms. The sequence of events begins with a stimulus—your husband's behavior. If his behavior patterns, which you have come to know so well, conformed to your expectations, there would have been no alarm, no threat, no anxiety. In fact, when people behave precisely as we expect them to, we often take no notice at all. We do not receive or attend to all the stimuli in our environment, but only to those most relevant to our vital interests. When your husband suddenly begins acting in strange and unpredictable ways, you notice. You evaluate the uncertainty and inappropriateness as dangerous, a threat to the well-being of your family. You told yourself "something is wrong with Lou." You view this threat as a serious one, and you feel vulnerable because you don't know how to meet it. It is too far outside the range of your prior experience for you to have developed strategies to deal with this type of threat. However, our evolutionary history has provided us with automatic and primal reactions to danger that are designed as survival mechanisms to provide protection under conditions of such serious threat. We refer to these reactions as the *fight-or-flight response* after the physiological changes that are the most dramatic components. Some of these changes produced the symptoms you experienced in the car— racing heart, rapid breathing, increased muscle tension, and sweating.

You said this was a survival mechanism, designed to protect us from danger. I don't understand how these changes protected me from anything. They made me feel awful.

Remember, we said the fight-or-flight response is an ancient and primitive one. When humans lived in caves and jungles, sudden threats from wild beasts elicited a cluster of physiologic responses, such as those you just described. These responses maximized the physical strength or speed required to outfight or outrun a powerful predator. Under those conditions, the increased heart rate, breathing and muscle tension were survival mechanisms. Today, we rarely face such sudden threats to our existence. However, the response mechanism is still part of our genetic make-up. It is called forth by an actual physical threat, or, more often, by a perception of threat that poses no immediate danger to your survival. Your husband's unexpected behavior was just such a perceived threat and the fight-or-flight response was activated. But neither speed nor physical strength is likely to prove effective in dealing with the problems posed by your husband's illness.

What about the feeling of nervousness, always being on edge, as if doom were about to strike?

This is the emotional component, which we call anxiety. It can also be a compelling and unpleasant experience.

I'll say! Is it helpful in any way?

Up to a point, yes. Emotional arousal can motivate you to seek options, implement problem-solving strategies, take timely actions. But beyond that point, excessive emotional arousal begins to interfere with adaptive behavior. Anxiety about Lou prompted you to seek medical advice. Excessive anxiety in the car nearly led you to an accident.

Chronic anxiety is another way in which anxiety becomes dysfunctional. By this we mean remaining geared up for defensive action after the danger has passed, or remaining so sensitized to danger that you see threat where none exists. When this happens, you overreact to innocuous or mildly threatening situations as if they portended immediate disaster.

I think that's what is happening. I always feel keyed up and on edge. As I told you, even when Lou seems O.K., I worry.

Let's talk about worry, then. It is another component in the basic survival mechanism we all share—the cognitive, or thinking, component. What do you worry about most?

It's hard to sort out. I worry about everything, all the time. It seems like everything I think about triggers anxiety.

The statement you just made demonstrates a typical distortion that tends to creep into our thinking at times of stress. It is called overgeneralization, and it is part of the vicious cycle by which anxiety breeds more anxiety. While it is probably true that you worry much of the time about many things, it is hardly likely that you worry all the time about everything. Wouldn't you agree?

Yes, I suppose I am exaggerating. But when I feel so upset, it's hard for me to put my thoughts into words.

This is another illustration of how high levels of anxiety can interfere with adaptive behavior, especially a complex and cognitively demanding task like verbalizing your thoughts.

Initially, your anxiety was probably activated by the sheer mismatch between what you expected of Lou and what you got. Such a discrepancy from accepted and appropriate standards of behavior seemed to you very threatening. Your inner dialogue probably went something like: "Uh oh, something is very wrong with Lou, and I don't know what to do about it. And I am terrified."

Perhaps. But I don't really remember thinking anything in particular—just feeling terrified.

That's because the emotional and physiological components are so dramatic and unpleasant. They tend to get noticed and remembered while the thoughts, the worries, that triggered them get overlooked and forgotten. But it is important for us to be aware of our thoughts, because by changing them we can regulate our feelings. For example, do you recall what you told us about the first time Lou repeated the same question over and over?

Yes, I thought he was joking, and I didn't like it. I got annoyed.

That's right. You got annoyed, not scared or panicked. That's because of what you told yourself—your thoughts. You probably told yourself something like, "I wish Lou wouldn't act like such a wise guy."

True. But that isn't what I thought when he didn't know who I was.

No. Then you knew something was seriously amiss.

I remember now. I did tell myself something like you suggested earlier. I thought, "What if Lou is going crazy? I could never handle that."

So you panicked because you felt threatened by a danger with which you thought you could not possibly cope. This belief, and others, are likely to continue to generate feelings of anxiety until you learn to challenge them.

Others?

Yes. Now that you have taken the first steps to find out what is wrong with Lou and what might be done about it, it is likely that other worries, other threatening thoughts, will occur to you, such as what changes Lou might show next.

I do worry about that.

This is called *anticipatory* anxiety, because it has to do with events that have not happened and may not ever happen. To help you keep your levels of anxiety manageable, we'd better identify these thoughts and help you challenge them.

Challenge them? How?

By reevaluating their likelihood, their awfulness, and your ability to deal with the threats they represent.

Why do I have to identify my worries? Just thinking about trying to do that makes me uncomfortable. I'd rather you helped me to forget about my worries, not to dwell on them.

We don't recommend dwelling on problems. In fact, one dictionary definition of worry is "to torment oneself with disturbing thoughts." But we don't think avoidance will help you in the long run either.

Why not? You just said some of what I worry about may never happen.

But some of what you anticipate probably will occur and will have to be dealt with. Even if that doesn't happen, avoidance of troublesome thoughts or situations actually breeds more anxiety. This is the vicious cycle we alluded to earlier.

How does it work?

When you avoid, rather than face, something unpleasant or uncomfortable, you tend to overestimate or "awfulize" both the threat and the discomfort it arouses. You tend also to minimize your own ability to deal with both, thus increasing the sense of vulnerability to harm that triggers anxiety in the first place. The result is usually more frequent and more intense anxiety, more things perceived as threatening, more avoidance, and a constricted life. Eventually, this could have serious consequences for your self-esteem and emotional well-being.

O.K. One of the things I worry about is Lou becoming violent. As I told you, I don't know much about AD, if that's what this is. But I have heard of cases where people go berserk and hurt their loved ones without realizing what they are doing. Are you telling me this won't happen?

No. Unfortunately, we can't guarantee that Lou won't behave violently. Nor can we assure you that he won't accidentally injure himself or others if he does have a progressive dementing disease. If he doesn't, then these problems will not materialize. But let's suppose he does. Would it be adaptive for you to ignore the possibility? Or to worry about it?

No. But what else is there to do?

There is appropriate concern. Recognizing and accepting that unpleasant and dangerous events may occur is adaptive. It leads you to make contingency plans to minimize the likelihood of such events, or to deal with them if they occur. You may, for example, have to call the police if you are physically threatened, so it would be practical for you to know the number of your local precinct. In addition, ask your physician for a mild sedative to have on hand just in case. But to dwell endlessly and fruitlessly on how awful it would be if this happened is a waste of time and energy. It generates anxiety rather than concern. It drains you and makes you less efficient.

So, if I acknowledge the possibility of unpleasant things happening and think of some options in case they do, then I don't have to spend so much time anticipating them.

Precisely. If you refrain from "awfulizing" in advance about events that may be unpleasant, you won't get so anxious so often. And remember, there is no law that says you must come up with a terrific solution to all problems.

O.K. I can tell myself that it is all right to call the police if I have to. But there are other things.

Such as?

I worry about Lou deteriorating—you know, becoming disheveled and unkempt-looking, refusing to wash, becoming incontinent, smelling bad. I remember visiting a great-aunt once in a nursing home. I was just a kid, but I never forgot how the residents looked. To this day, I can't stand to look at deteriorated elderly people. I can't stand to think about Lou getting that way.

What you are describing now is *discomfort* anxiety. It is, in effect, anxiety about anxiety. What you remember so vividly from this childhood experience is basically similar to what you recall from the incident in the car when Lou didn't know who you were; namely, how you *felt*. Those feelings were very uncomfortable. You didn't like them. But you did stand them, didn't you?

Just barely. I remember that I had bad dreams for a long time. I was afraid that my parents would get that way, too.

Yes, and you carried that childhood fear throughout your life. Your past anxiety about your parents has now been rekindled in the form of anticipatory anxiety about Lou's condition. Lou's condition will undoubtedly deteriorate. You perceive this as a threat with which you will not be able to cope.

How does this anticipatory anxiety help you to cope better with the daily problems that you have to face now?

It doesn't. In fact, it makes it harder. So what do I do?

Tell yourself that feeling anxious and uncomfortable is not pleasant, but it won't kill you. Tell yourself that you *can* stand it even if you don't like it.

It seems like there are two parts to my worries—one, what will happen to Lou and what will I do about it; and two, what will happen to me, and can I stand the way I feel?

That's a good observation. Let's try to come up with more rational and effective self-talk for both parts. What can you tell yourself about Lou's potential deterioration and what you, as a caregiver, can do for him?

I can learn as much as possible about his disease. I can stop anticipating catastrophes. I can tell myself that unpleasant things may happen, and I'll do the best I can if they do.

Good. Remind yourself that you may not be able to come up with terrific solutions that will make everything all right, nor do you have to. If this is AD, then there are no perfect answers here, no happy ending before the last commercial. And you can accept the fact that you will feel uncomfortable and even anxious from time to time, because you are in a threatening situation. You do not have to make yourself anxious about having anxiety. The feelings are unpleasant but not dangerous, and they pass. You can help yourself to feel less vulnerable by reminding yourself that you do have coping skills and can learn others, that you can seek help and support from others, and that there are people out there who have dealt with the tragedy of AD and survived. So can you!

———•———

My mother was diagnosed as having Alzheimer's disease several years ago. She lives with my sister and brother-in-law now, and I try to visit once a month or so. Whenever I do, I find I have trouble sleeping at night. I toss and turn, I have nightmares, and I feel uptight for several days afterward. I can't stand feeling that way, so it's getting harder and harder for me to push myself to make that visit. I'm tempted to avoid it altogether. Needless to say, that makes me feel rotten.

You are describing what we call discomfort anxiety—anxiety about feeling anxious and uncomfortable. It produces a strong tendency to avoid situations in which you have those feelings.

I do have those feelings every time I visit Mom. But I don't want to avoid her, so what do I do?

Discomfort anxiety is sometimes called secondary anxiety because it emerges *after* one already feels anxious about something else. You can deal with the problem in two ways. First, reduce the discomfort anxiety directly by changing what you are telling yourself about the unpleasant feelings you have. When you don't get so upset over having them, this will counteract the tendency to avoid. Second, identify what triggered the initial anxiety in the first place so that you feel less uncomfortable when you do visit your mother.

Let's start with the secondary anxiety. Have you been telling yourself that you can't stand the discomfort, the sleepless nights and tension you experience after visiting your mother?

Yes, I have.

But you do stand it, don't you?

Not very well.

True. Nevertheless, you are here, and you are standing it. You could stand it better if you told yourself something different.

Like what? That it's perfectly fine for me to be a nervous wreck once a month?

No, that would be inappropriate. To label yourself a "nervous wreck" because you occasionally feel nervous is to commit the error of overgeneralization. Also, it is not adaptive to pretend that you like a situation that you deplore. A better self-statement would be, "I don't like feeling anxious and uncomfortable, but it won't kill me. I can stand even what I dislike."

I could tell myself that. I can see how that would help me deal with the reluctance to go see my mother.

Right. If you don't "awfulize" your feelings, there's no incentive to avoid them. Now, tell us what you think about when you visit. This will help us identify the initial triggers of your anxiety.

I keep remembering my grandmother. She died many years ago—before most people had ever heard of AD. They said she was senile. But she seemed to be so much like my mother is now. I mean, she did the same strange things, like forgetting who we were, who she was, stuffing food into dresser drawers, accusing people of stealing her things, wandering off, and prowling the house all night. I'm pretty sure she had AD. Now my mother has it. I wonder what will happen to me—will I go the same route? Sometimes I can almost see myself in that condition, and it terrifies me.

Obviously, the image of yourself being afflicted with AD is a frightening one. This potential threat, which you can do nothing about, generates the initial anxiety that interferes with sleep and makes you tense. Anxiety is triggered by threats we feel unable to meet. It can be alleviated by reevaluating the degree of danger or our ability to meet it.

In this case, you can reevaluate the degree of risk to yourself by examining the research. There is some evidence of familial clusters that suggests that at least some forms of AD may have a genetic component. But it is far from clear that this is the case in general. Even in those families at risk, not all members develop AD. There are many theories about the etiology, or cause, of AD, some implicating viruses or toxic substances, others multiple factors acting together, but the jury is still out on this one. There may be an "Alzheimer's gene," carried by a small percentage of the total population. But we can't identify those people, nor can we say which of them will actually develop the disease. The risk appears to be higher in families where AD often occurs before age sixty and afflicts both parents and siblings. Your family does not fit that profile, and so the risk to you is probably not different from anyone in the general population.

That's reassuring. But I can't get rid of that frightening picture of myself in a deteriorated condition.

Let's see if you can change it. Try to see yourself in your later years as vigorous, healthy, and active— playing with your grandchildren, or perhaps enjoying sports, hobbies, or another of your favorite activities. Close your eyes and use all your senses to sharpen and make more vivid this positive image.

I can do it.

Does it help?

Yes, it does.

This is an excellent general anti-anxiety technique. We recommend you practice it and use it often.

———•—•———

I've been caring for my husband for seven years. He was seventy-three when they diagnosed his condition as AD, and I'm three years younger, so as you can see, we're not that young anymore. Caring for Phil has not been a bed of roses for me, but I've managed. Unfortunately, it's taken a toll on me. Lately I feel like my strength is giving out, and I'm worried what will become of Phil if anything happens to me—if I become incapacitated or die.

What do you think will happen?

I don't know. Phil is completely dependent on me. We have no children. There is a younger brother, but he lives in a different part of the country, and they've never been particularly close. I'm positive he wouldn't assume the responsibility for Phil's care.

What other options have you?

I have no options. I keep thinking of Phil left all alone here to fend for himself. He can't dress or feed himself without my help—he'd starve. It would be horrible. I can feel myself getting upset just talking about it. And I dwell on it.

To have concern about your husband's welfare should you die first is realistic. But to dwell on it—to worry constantly—is maladaptive. None of us has a guarantee of continued good health. None of us knows for certain that we will continue to be able to discharge our responsibilities, whether to dependent children, dependent spouses, or dependent parents. So we make contingency plans, such as purchasing health, life, accident, or disability insurance, writing wills, setting up trusts or guardianships, or entering into less formal agreements with friends or relatives. Then, having done what we can, we go on with our lives.

That's fine for those other problems. But as I told you, in my situation, there are no options.

There may not be any perfect solutions, or even any good options, but that is hardly the same as having no options whatsoever. This is another example of the cognitive error we are all susceptible to, namely, all-or-nothing or black-white thinking: if things aren't terrific, then they must be terrible, with no in-betweens. How does this kind of thinking help you to accomplish your primary goal, to maximize the quality of Phil's care?

Actually, it doesn't help. I know that, but I can't seem to do anything about it. I try to think of possible solutions, but all that happens is I feel more and more anxious.

That's because you are putting the cart before the horse. You are trying to come up with practical solutions before emotional solutions. A more effective strategy is to cope with the emotion first. Then you can seek and find better options for your practical problem.

O.K. So how do I do that?

Let's examine some of the things you have been telling yourself about dying before your husband, because this is how you make yourself upset and anxious.

You make it sound as if I had a choice. I don't make myself upset—it's the awful situation I'm in.

We believe that you do have a choice as to how you respond emotionally to your admittedly difficult and unpleasant situation.

How else could I possibly respond? With joy?

No. That would be equally inappropriate and maladaptive. But so is worry—torturing yourself with frightening thoughts. It is these thoughts that produce the anxiety and upset, and these thoughts can be changed if you work at it.

For example, you have been telling yourself that Phil is totally dependent upon you, that if you abandoned him—for that is how you see it—his fate would be horrible, namely starvation.

That's true.

Not quite. What you have been telling yourself is "awfulized" and overgeneralized. It is true that Phil is dependent, but is he dependent solely upon you? Is it only you who can stand between him and starvation?

Yes. I have already told you that there is nobody else.

You have indicated that there is no immediate relative who will assume Phil's care. Is that the only option? What about agencies and institutions that society provides for the care of dependent persons without family?

You're talking about nursing homes. I visited one. I couldn't stand for Phil to wind up in such a place.

Some nursing homes leave much to be desired in

quality of care. But does that mean *all* are equally inadequate?

No. It's just that I never envisioned such an outcome. I always assumed I'd be able to care for him until the end.

Yes, and in your view, that was the best, the ideal, way to care for him. But now you are facing the fact that ideal solutions aren't always possible. To continue to demand that they should be is maladaptive. It generates emotional upset and dissipates energy that could better be applied to finding an acceptable, if not ideal, solution. Once you can accept the best you can do within the limits of the possible—even if that is far from what you had hoped for—then your emotional response will be appropriate concern, and you will be free to seek and find a solution you can live with.

Instead of Saying . . .	**Tell Yourself . . .**
What will I do about the awful things in store for me?	I will handle unpleasant things if they happen as best I can. I don't have to anticipate catastrophes.
I can't possibly care for my relative if he gets worse.	My relative undoubtedly will get worse. I will do the best I can for him, and it won't be perfect.
I can't stand feeling so anxious and upset.	Feelings of anxiety are uncomfortable, but they won't kill me. I can stand it.
What if the same disease happens to me?	It is impossible for anyone to foretell the future, including one's future health. I can live a healthy, satisfying lifestyle, one day at a time.

Instead of Saying . . .	**Tell Yourself . . .**
I can't possibly cope with this.	I do have coping skills for this situation, and I can learn new ones.
I dread what the future will bring.	The future may be very painful. But catastrophizing about it today won't help resolve today's problems or ward off tomorrow's.

CHAPTER 10

Depression: Life Is So Bleak

I have been feeling pretty low lately. I've lost weight. I don't sleep very well. I'm tired all the time. Nothing interests me. And I find it hard to drag myself out of bed in the morning. I had a complete checkup, and the doctor didn't find a thing wrong with me. He said I'm depressed.

Sounds like it. How long have you felt this way?

I've been aware of this exhausted feeling about two months. But, in retrospect, I would say it's been coming on gradually for quite a while.

Have you ever felt this down for any length of time before?

No, not that I can remember.

Has anything happened in your life, any big change?

Yes. When Jerry was diagnosed as having AD—about three years ago. That was a big shock. I knew something was wrong—I knew it for quite a while. At times he didn't seem like himself—forgetful, sometimes angry over the strangest things. I assumed it was tension because he was facing involuntary retirement at sixty-five, in two years. But when he insisted that we go visit his mother, who had died fifteen years ago, I could no longer pretend that this was something I could ignore. That's when we went through all the examinations until we were told that it was AD.

Do you think that your depression was triggered by that turn of events?

Probably. We had to make some big changes in our lives as a result.

Such as?

For one thing, Jerry had to quit work sooner than we anticipated. For another, I had to give up my job to stay at home with him.

You see, soon after the children left, I took a brush-up course and went back to work. I'm a bookkeeper. I finally worked my way into a good job in a good office. I enjoyed my work very much. And the money helped us live very comfortably.

But Jerry's illness progressed, as I was told it would, and I realized that he could no longer be left alone. I didn't want to leave him with a stranger. So I decided to stay home and devote myself to him.

And how do you feel, staying home?

I know it was the right decision. In fact, the only decision I could make. But . . .

Yes?

Everything has changed. I feel that life has come to an end.

For Jerry?

For Jerry and for me. I feel that there's nothing to get out of bed for. Except that Jerry needs me. So I force myself up to take care of him. That's my day.

In what specific way has life changed?

We used to go out. We went to theaters, concerts, vacations. We visited friends. Now we just stay home. Very few people come. I don't entertain anymore. Life is so bleak and depressing.

It's certainly very sad that Jerry has succumbed to this serious dementing illness. And there's no doubt that this significantly narrows your options. Life has become very constricted for you. But do you feel that allowing yourself to become depressed about it has helped you to see what options you do, in fact, have?

Allowing myself to become depressed? I don't allow myself to become depressed. I just do. I don't see how it can be otherwise. Wouldn't anyone in my situation be depressed?

Although most people having a mate with AD feel very sad, not all become depressed. There's a difference between realistic sadness and depression.

What's the difference?

Sadness is one component of depression. But sadness alone doesn't become the overwhelming, predominant mood, and it doesn't exclude other emotions. Depression does.

Sadness is a specific emotional response to a specific sad situation, such as the one you are now in. Realistic sadness leaves room for other emotions, such as happiness and pleasure, to light your hours or your days. It is part of your total emotional repertory. Feeling sad does not interfere with your ability to make rational decisions and make rational choices.

Depression, on the other hand, becomes pervasive. It's an all-or-nothing state of mind. It may be triggered by an external event, such as a loss, or a death, but it is shaped and sustained by your own evaluation of that event. Jerry's illness was the spark that set you on the path to depression. But what you say to yourself about it determines whether you will feel realistically sad or whether you will feel depressed.

Depression doesn't just automatically happen as a result of a set of noxious circumstances. It comes about as a result of your view of yourself, your world, your situation, your ability to cope. It is an emotional over-response to what you perceive as a crushing blow. Since the evaluation of your situation resides within you, not in the event itself, it is within your power to change that.

I don't understand how I can change that. Please explain.

The best way to help you sort out the ways in which you depress yourself is to examine your various beliefs and assumptions and deal with them one at a time. If your assumptions about your world, and your place in it, are illogical and unrealistic, the chances are that you will become not just sad, but depressed. So let's deal with them separately, to see how we can correct them and bring them more in line with reality.

It feels like a part of me has been lost. Maybe there's some truth to the old joking reference to one's mate as "my better half." And that half is gone—and not gone.

Can you spell out what is gone?

I have no one to talk to—the ordinary bits and pieces of daily living. I read something in the paper, and I want to comment on it. I see something on TV, and he sits next to me, and I know that it's just meaningless moving images to him. I can't even complain about anything to him—an incorrect bill, or the fact that I haven't heard from the children in a week. Nothing. All I get is a blank stare. Or anger. I can no longer understand him. Or he, me. I feel that I've lost my husband. And yet he's there, but only for me to take care of. It's all so hopeless.

Yes, that is a very deep-seated and meaningful loss. Where formerly there was mutual exchange and mutual understanding, now you face uncertainty, ambiguity, and chaotic behavior.

In many ways, this is harder to bear than death. Death is open, it's acknowledged, it's final. It has rituals to mark its finality. And society generally rallies around the bereaved person.

There are no rituals for the death of the mind. And society is generally either callous or rejecting.

Some of the depression you are now experiencing is undoubtedly bereavement. That's understandable. It's a mourning process for a lost loved one, or a lost life with a loved one who is, as you say, gone but still here. Unfortunately, after thirty-five years of marriage, it's necessary to begin to separate yourself from him, emotionally and intellectually, while he is still with you physically.

How can I do that?

By changing your expectation of him. That is, by expecting that at times he will be angry at what seems to you to be trivial, that he will be rejecting when you think you deserve praise, that he will be unpredictable and strange. In other words, by not expecting him to be the husband that he once was, or the husband that you want him to be. And, because he isn't the husband that he once was, and never will be, you feel that life is hopeless. That is one of your illogical and unrealistic assumptions.

Why is it illogical and unrealistic?

Because, in actuality, Jerry's illness *is* hopeless, in the sense that it is irreversible and deteriorative. So, to see it as hopeless is realistic. But your life is not hopeless. It has changed in many important ways. But that is not the same as saying that life for you is hopeless.

What hope is there for me? I look into the future, and I see nothing but darkness.

You are confusing two issues. One is the outlook for Jerry's life. As we know, there is, at present, no hope for a turnabout in his illness. Even if science should find an effective treatment, it will undoubtedly come too late to help anyone as far gone as Jerry seems to be. There is no hope that he will ever be able to participate in a cultural, intellectual, or social life with you. There is no hope for a full and rich life of shared experiences with you. But does that mean that there is no hope for enjoyment of concerts, theater, and friends, apart from him?

How? I've never done anything without him. I don't know if I can. I got married at twenty-one, and I've always seen myself as part of a couple.

Is being part of a couple the same as being half a person?

No, but I guess that's how I've always seen myself. And now that the other half is not functioning, I don't know who or what I am.

Unfortunately, most women have been raised to believe that they absolutely need a man in order to be whole persons. While most women would agree that sharing one's life with a loving and understanding man is desirable, that is not the same as saying that without one, a woman is just half a person. When you look at yourself as half a person, you are putting yourself down. And every time that you put yourself down about anything, you depress yourself.

But we live in a coupled world. And many people look upon a woman alone as a pariah, a social outcast. A man alone is seen as a social asset.

That's true, to a great extent. Although, fortunately, that's changing. But why do you have to accept the judgment of people who are narrow-minded and bigoted? When you refuse to accept their judgment, you realize that it is they, not you, who have a problem. When you accept yourself as a whole person, you will feel freer to act in your own best interest.

So, just keep telling yourself, "It would be great to turn the clock back and still be part of a functioning couple, but that's not the way it is—or will be."

Yes, but . . . If you are suggesting that I go places without Jerry, that's just not possible.

Why not?

Because it wouldn't be right.

What's wrong with that?

I feel that I would be betraying Jerry.

In what way?

My place is by his side. For me to go out would mean hiring someone to stay with him. When my children were small, I always stayed with them. I never hired sitters while I went gallivanting around. I didn't go back to work until they were grown. When I quit my job to stay home with Jerry, I decided that my place was at his side, taking care of him. I would feel guilty doing otherwise.

What would you be guilty of, if you went out once in a while? "Dereliction of duty?"

Dereliction of duty sounds so legal and like a formal charge. No, not exactly dereliction of duty. I would just feel guilty.

Well, if you're not really guilty of any serious offense, why make yourself feel gulity?

Because my job is to take care of him.

Twenty-four hours a day? Seven days a week?

I see no choice.

You do have a choice. It's not an all-or-nothing choice. It's not a choice between neglecting Jerry or spending all your time out on the town. It's not even a choice between submerging yourself totally in Jerry's care or going out once in a while.

It's a choice between seeing yourself as a person whose sole function in life is the welfare of other persons, or as a person entitled to some autonomy, some independent existence, some right to open an occasional window on the world for herself—even under the most trying circumstances.

Obviously, this is a difficult choice for many women. So many women judge themselves—and are judged by others—by their level of devotion to, and level of commitment to, other people. While this is often admirable, insofar as it provides the warmth and the caring that women bring to their relationships, if

carried to extremes it also paves the way for depression. That's one reason why so many more women than men are depressed.

When you say, "It's my job to take care of him," this is a job description written by you. Since you wrote the job description, you can rewrite it and include some breathing space for yourself. But first, it's necessary to convince yourself that you're entitled to it. You are entitled to it, not because you have earned any special dispensation, but because you are a human being with needs and wants independent of your husband's needs and wants. To deny yourself totally is one avenue to depression. Remind yourself of this frequently and vigorously. In other words, change what you have been telling yourself.

Once you have convinced yourself that you are entitled to some space, you will then be able to define, for yourself, how much. And you won't feel guilty about taking it.

But wouldn't that be selfish?

Selfishness means indulging in your own interests without regard for the interests and welfare of others. The opposite of selfishness would be self-effacement, or total neglect of one's own interests and welfare. Again, to counterpose the one against the other is to indulge in all-or-nothing thinking. All-or-nothing thinking, as we see over and over again, is a common fallacy that pervades much of the maladaptive cognitive processes underlying depression.

Then what would be an adaptive choice?

Something in between. Let's call it rational self-care, or self-assertion, within the context of suitable care for Jerry. And you will have to decide for yourself what your own requirements are.

I don't seem to be able to decide anything anymore.

Like what?

I used to be very competent. I know I was competent on my job and at home. Now it seems that I can't do anything right.

What don't you do right?

Everything.

Everything is pretty broad. Please explain.

Whatever I do for Jerry seems to be wrong. He blows up at the least little thing. Whatever I cook is no good. Whatever I buy is the wrong thing. On the rare occasions when I ask people to visit, they're always people he "hates."

Then what you're really saying is that everything that you do for Jerry meets with his disapproval. Is that right?

Yes.

Is Jerry the best judge of your competence?

No, not really.

Then why do you say that you can't do anything right when what you really mean is that Jerry doesn't approve of most things that you do for him?

And since you admit that he is not a very good judge of events nowadays, why do you accept his opinion as valid? And allow that opinion to depress you?

It's not only what Jerry says. . . . I actually don't seem to be able to do anything right. That's the way it is now.

Tell me one thing that you do with a fair degree of probability that it will turn out right.

I can't think of anything.

How about making a cup of tea? With a tea bag?

Of course, I can do that. Everyone can make a cup of tea—with a tea bag.

Can Jerry?

No. Not anymore. In fact, last week he took a tea bag out of the package and asked me what it was for.

So "everyone" minus Jerry can make a cup of tea. That reduces the category from "everyone" to "everyone minus one." And now we know that you don't do everything wrong. Only everything minus making a cup of tea.

That's silly.

It may sound silly, but it tells us something.

What does it tell us?

It tells us again that you indulge in all-or-nothing thinking. What we call overgeneralization. If I can't do some things right, I can't do anything right. And overgeneralization can get you into a pretty depressed mood. Black or white with nothing in between.

Now that we have established that you can make a cup of tea—with a tea bag—what else can you do right?

I can't think of anything.

Who handles the family finances? Balances the checkbook?

I do.

And do the books balance?

Yes, of course. I'm a bookkeeper.

Then we have two areas of competence: making a cup of tea, and handling the family finances. It's very likely that you can do lots more than this competently. But you don't allow yourself to see the positives. You focus exclusively on the negatives!

You see, when you feel down about yourself, you see only the down side. Your black mood colors the events in your life and makes them appear all negative—with no redeeming features. This works two ways. You say, "Because I do everything badly, I'm no good," and "Because I'm no good, I do everything badly." So you fence yourself in and set yourself up for a self-fulfilling prophecy. That is, you say to yourself, "Everything will inevitably turn out wrong." And in your negative mood, it's likely that whatever does turn out not to your liking, or to Jerry's liking, or is less than perfect, will prove your point, namely that you are really not a worthwhile person.

What can I do about it?

In the first place, stop rating yourself. People aren't rateable. If, on a scale of one to ten, something you do rates a ten, and some other endeavor earns no points, then are you a five? Obviously, you can't average your good and bad performances and come up with a rating of yourself as a person. So it's wise and realistic to look at yourself as a person with good, bad, and so-so abilities and traits. Then you won't put yourself down if Jerry criticizes you. You can then try to change those behaviors that you yourself don't like and accept the totality of you as a person.

If your best efforts on Jerry's behalf don't meet with his approval, in what way does this reflect on you, rather than on his judgment?

It doesn't really reflect on me. But I feel that I have let him down. It's not just what he says. But I feel that I'm a failure.

In what way have you let him down?

If I weren't such a washout most of the time, I could think of ways to help him.

The lethargy, which you call a washout, is just a symptom of your depression. Are you blaming yourself for feeling this way?

Yes. I feel that if I could pull myself together, he would not be going downhill the way he is doing. I feel so helpless.

Has anyone ever told you that it was within your power to alter—or even slow down—the course of Jerry's illness?

No.

Then don't you think that it's a little grandiose on your part to think that you are responsible for his deterioration?

You just told me that I was putting myself down. Now you tell me that I'm being grandiose. Aren't you contradicting yourself? Which is it?

Both. They're two sides of the same coin. And neither is rooted in reality. So what we would like you to do is to learn to think more realistically.

When you put yourself down, you heap blame on yourself for not measuring up to some standard of behavior that you set for yourself. Then you set that goal at an unrealistic and untenable level. Since you can't reach that goal, you then blame yourself and put yourself down for having failed. And you feel blameworthy and call yourself a failure.

So let's see how that pertains to your evaluation of your own behavior, your belief that you have failed your husband. When you imply that you should be able to prevent Jerry's deterioration, you are setting an impossible goal based on wishful thinking, not reality. Since your husband's deterioration is obviously due to a brain process outside of your control, you are doomed to feeling that you failed him by not being able to change its course.

Then the seemingly logical conclusion that you draw is that you are no good, a failure. So you see that both your grandiosity and your self-putdown and your self-blame stem from the same illogical evaluation of events. If, more realistically, you could say to yourself, "His illness is unfortunate. I can't control or change it. I can only do what I can to make him as comfortable as I know how. And my knowledge and experience of this are both extremely limited," you would feel less depressed than you do.

It's wise to realize that you are indeed helpless in this one very critical area of your life. You are helpless to make a healthy person out of the demented man who is your husband. There is no way to change that. But does that mean that you are a failure?

I guess not.

No, because to call yourself a failure is, again, an overgeneralization. A failure is one who fails. We might qualify that definition by saying that a failure is one who always fails. That leaves no room for success in any aspect of one's life. Do you think that's true of you? Obviously not! We have already established that you can make a cup of tea, keep the family accounts, and, undoubtedly, see to Jerry's needs and comforts. Yet, because your best efforts to improve Jerry's condition have failed, you have branded yourself a failure. Then you've blamed yourself, felt guilty, and condemned yourself as worthless.

Now, you may have made mistakes—as we all do—but in what way does that make you worthless? Suppose that your kitchen sink had a leaky faucet. Would you consider your house worthless?

No, of course not.

It wouldn't be perfect. But to condemn the house because of a leaky faucet would be a case of overgeneralization, wouldn't it?

Yes. But you would fix the faucet.

And you can fix your own overgeneralizations about yourself.

How?

Not by calling the plumber, but by modifying some aspects of your thinking.

How?

By telling yourself two things: One, I am human and fallible, and prone to make mistakes; and two, I am a worthwhile person, even if I have made mistakes.

And if I tell myself this, I will no longer be depressed? Just like that?

That would be a starting point in overcoming your depression. It's not all of it.

You see, change involves two difficult steps. The first is giving up your old habit of heaping blame upon yourself, and the other is to institute the new habit of unconditional self-acceptance.

Old habits of thought, like old habits of penmanship or any other learned skill, become deeply ingrained. Patterns of neural activity are formed in your brain and nervous system. These, once established, maintain the habit and result in automatic functioning. For example, once you've learned to drive a car, you do so automatically, without thinking about each step. The same with old, well-learned—or what we call overlearned—responses. Old thoughts occur spontaneously, as if from nowhere, when, in fact, they are learned responses, practiced by repetition since early childhood. "I am no good if . . .", "I am worthless if . . .", "I am guilty if I did—or if I didn't . . .", "I don't deserve to . . ." These negative self-evaluations have been taught to us by well-meaning parents, teachers, and friends. They are generally instilled as a means of social control during the long course of teaching children to behave according to the accepted standard of society. It is the child, then, who often overgeneralizes and transforms these negative learned precepts into condemnation of himself.

At the same time that you actively work against your old negative habits of self-condemnatory thinking, it's important to practice new habits of total self-acceptance. And that takes conscious effort and practice.

What kind of practice?

Let's say that you once learned to type, many years ago, using your two index fingers—the hunt-and-peck method. You managed to get along on a limited basis. But at some point, you reached a dead end. You could never get a job involving typing skills. Your limited method handicapped you. So you decided to learn to type, using all ten fingers. Your old habit continually got in your way. It was hard to give up. You thought it was the more "natural" way. But it wasn't more natural; it was simply an overlearned habit. And because it was overlearned, it seemed spontaneous and natural. So you had to work triply hard, and consciously, to overcome the maladaptive old fingering, while you practiced the new. At the same time, the old habit kept reasserting itself as if it had a will of its own. You felt more comfortable with the old fingering, even if it became a roadblock to improvement. But if you wanted a better job, with a better future, you had to give up the old habit and make the new one become automatic, spontaneous, and natural.

Now let's apply this analogy to one aspect of your current problem: your tendency to put yourself down when events do not turn out to your liking. "I'm no good" is a thought that seems logical, spontaneous, and natural, when in fact it is an overlearned, maladaptive habit of responding. Since it is a learned response, it can be unlearned and replaced with more adaptive self-evaluations.

Such as?

Such as unconditional self-acceptance. Every time you say to yourself, "I am no good," stop and say, "I am human and worthwhile." Keep repeating this until you fully believe it and it replaces the former self-derogatory self-statements. That's what we mean by unconditional self-acceptance.

Does that mean that I automatically approve of everything I do?

No, it means that you accept yourself, with your flaws—which we all have—and your good points— which it's wise to recognize. It means examining your flaws realistically and honestly and making changes when possible. It means accepting mistakes as part of the human condition. It means taking responsibility for your own actions, and not taking responsibility for events that you cannot control.

Well, if I practice new habits of thinking, and if I accept myself unconditionally, as you suggest, and if I don't take Jerry's criticism of me or his outbursts personally, that still leaves me feeling like I'm out in the cold and shivering.

What do you mean?

When you see your husband slowly slipping away from you; and when other people who, you thought were close to you, now hardly ever call you—what keeps you going?

These two questions have one element in common; that is *relatedness*. It's when relatedness, or a sense of connection to other people, is lost, that one feels "out in the cold and shivering."

The input that you normally expected from Jerry is gone. The old give and take that balances a relationship and sustains it no longer exists. Your relationship now is one of give, but do not take. Your world, the one based on mutual exchange, has collapsed. That leaves you angry, resentful, and "shivering."

The bonds of old social connections, too, often weaken, just when you need them most as stable anchors in a shifting world. And that is largely because few people know how to cope with a frightening and largely unknown disease—a disease that has only recently acquired a name.

It is, after all, a disease of advancing age that until recently was believed to be an inevitable stage of life, on the road to death. So it appears threatening to most people.

No one wants to die young. And no one wants to live to old age if it means decline and dementia. Although we now know that only five percent of the population suffers from Alzheimer's Disease, in many people's minds longevity and dementia are synonymous. Therefore, many people, especially in our youth-oriented society, make themselves more comfortable by avoiding the declining and demented individual and her family.

This further adds to your sense of disconnectedness and isolation.

Then how can I best deal with this?

First of all, accept the reality that your husband is no longer available to you for emotional support. Accept the fact that—whatever the nature of your past relationship—it no longer rests on the same terms. Whatever he was to you before his illness, the overriding fact now is his dependency. This is inherent in his illness. This puts a double burden upon you: caring for him and maintaining your own life, apart from him.

As for your sense of social isolation, as your old friends withdraw from your circle, you are forced to face the fact that your life has changed in some basic ways. You are no longer a part of a couple, in a coupled society. But is this the end of the world?

Sometimes it seems like it.

Do you feel that you absolutely *need* these social relationships in order to come in out of the cold and stop "shivering"? Or is it that you *prefer* to have them continue as part of the social system you once enjoyed?

I don't understand.

Let's explain the difference between a need and a preference. If you say "I need these people," then you are making an absolute demand. You are, in effect, saying, "If I don't get what I need, then the world is cold and callous, and I must make myself absolutely miserable." And you will succeed in doing just that.

If, on the other hand, you say, "I prefer to keep my social circle intact," then you are making a realistic statement, not about the world, but about your own wishes and desires. Stating a preference, then, also implies that if it is not met, there are other choices that you might consider.

I did think I needed my old social structure, and I felt very angry and hurt to see it fall apart. I blamed Jerry for causing it, I blamed myself for seeing it happen, I blamed my friends for deserting me, and I blamed the world for being such a rotten place.

Instead of blaming anyone—Jerry, yourself, your friends, or the world—it's best to accept the change by saying, "I don't like what's happening. It's nobody's fault. It's just the way it is." Instead of saying, "I must have things the way they were," tell yourself "I would prefer if my old social life remained intact, but since it hasn't, let me look at what choices I do have."

What choices do I have?

There are practical steps to end your isolation. We will discuss these later on. But right now, let's continue to focus on your cognitive choices. By cognitive we mean the choice between giving yourself maladaptive messages that initiate, support, and deepen your depression, or adaptive ones that open the way for you to develop and enhance a more positive outlook, even as Jerry's illness worsens.

Such as?

Let's go back to what you said before about never getting any appreciation from Jerry for anything you do for him. It's true that we generally look for appreciation of our efforts. Appreciation from others is a very strong reinforcer. An infant reinforces us with a smile. A friend reinforces us by showing enjoyment of our company. A teacher reinforces us by giving us a good grade. An employer pays us for our efforts. Indifference, unjust criticism, and hostility put a damper on our efforts. Unfortunately, now that Jerry's care is so burdensome and painful, where will the reinforcement—the stroking—come from? Not from Jerry. He's unable to give it.

It surely won't come from his sister. She doesn't come over very often. The last time she came, she made some not-so-subtle remarks about the soup stains on Jerry's shirt. I had just changed it before lunch. I felt really down in the dumps when she left.

You felt down because you accepted her criticism as valid. You probably told yourself that she was right, that it's up to you to see that Jerry always looks perfectly neat and clean. And if he doesn't, that is a reflection on you. Self-blame again!

So, since few people who have not been exposed to AD fully understand the nature of this disease, it's wise not to expect much appreciation from them.

But you just said that we all expect reinforcement for our efforts.

Yes, that's true. And your reinforcement will come from the person in the best position to appreciate your efforts.

Who is that?

Yourself. Begin to appreciate yourself. Begin to give yourself positive messages. Begin to tell yourself, "Even if he didn't appreciate the walk we took, or the new sweater I bought him, or the lunch I prepared, I feel good about doing these things because it was right and because I know that I'm doing the best I can." Learning to praise yourself for your own positive deeds will free you from the often futile search for praise from others.

Isn't that being vain or boastful?

No, it's merely giving yourself recognition for your own competence in handling a very difficult situation. We are not suggesting that you go around telling everyone, "Look how great I am." We're not suggesting that you tell yourself, or anyone else, "I'm doing everything that can possibly be done for Jerry," because it's likely that more can be done. We are suggesting that you remind yourself that "That was well done," or, "That's O.K.," or "That's the best I can do"—or even, "That's O.K., even if I can do better." You don't have to perform at top efficiency. You are human, and like all other humans, you have your good days and your not-so-good days. Accept that.

And don't forget, when Jerry has a particularly crabby day, or series of days, to tell yourself, "There he goes again." That will serve to remind you that his crabbiness is due to his condition and not to any failure on your part.

When you learn to praise and appreciate yourself, you will still feel very alone, but much less lonely.

You say "Alone, but much less lonely." What's the difference between alone and lonely?

Alone is a statement of fact. You no longer have a husband with whom you can communicate. And you have lost some of your friends. So you are more alone than you have been in the past.

Loneliness is a feeling. It's a sense of sadness or desolation, a feeling of emptiness due to a lack of companionship. That's what you mean when you say that you feel "out in the cold and shivering." But when you recognize your own worth, and the worth of what you are doing, you become less dependent upon that companionship. You realize that it's certainly good to have the friendship of understanding people and the warmth of a caring husband, but you can survive without either. Feeling secure within yourself makes it possible to withstand the severe dislocations that your husband's illness precipitated. And it gives you the internal wherewithal to seek new relationships, new sources of satisfaction, and to develop new interests.

Depression isn't the result of just one set of illogical beliefs. It's a complex expression of an interlocking, and predominantly negative overlapping group of erroneous views of the world, of your situation, and of yourself.

In previous chapters, we discussed anger, self-pity, anxiety, and guilt. These are all negative emotions that, together with the pessimistic views discussed in this chapter, contribute to the depressive cluster.

Each person is different. You may experience each of these emotions to varying degrees. You may experience all at different times. Or you may experience some, but not others. It's highly unlikely, if you are a primary caregiver of an AD victim who is a significant person in your life, that you experience none of these negative emotions at any time.

Having a loved one with AD involves disappointments, unfulfilled hopes, frustrations, altered patterns of existence at a time when you are facing major adjustments in your life. But you don't have to become depressed.

Let's look at some of the illogical, maladaptive beliefs that are causing and maintaining your depression, and at some more adaptive beliefs with which you can replace them.

Instead of Saying . . .	Tell Yourself . . .
The future is dark, dreary, and hopeless.	My husband's future is hopeless. I can work to improve mine.
There's nothing left to live for.	I can explore my options and find new interests for myself.
I can't do anything right.	I'm not good at everything; I'm not poor at everything.
I'm helpless.	I'm helpless to change my husband's illness. I'm not helpless to change my life, while doing what I can for him.
It's not fair.	The world is not fair.
I must have other people's approval.	It's good to get other people's approval at times, but it's not *necessary* at any time.
I am a failure.	I may have failed at some endeavors, but that doesn't make me a failure.
This shouldn't have happened to me.	There are no "shoulds." This did happen to me.
I am miserable without a social life.	I can look for new friends and form new social networks.

Instead of Saying . . .	Tell Yourself . . .
The world is a pretty rotten place.	The world is not perfect. Neither am I. The world is not all bad. Neither am I.

CHAPTER 11

Stress: The Unity of Mind and Body

Lately, it seems I've been going to the doctor more and more often—and *I'm* the patient, not my husband. Even though Frank has had AD for a couple of years now, his physical health seems to be better than mine. Unlike me, he eats well, his heart is strong, and his blood pressure is normal. He almost never catches a cold, whereas I get every bug that goes around.

What does your doctor tell you?

She says I'm feeling the effects of all the stress I'm under, caring for Frank. That's why my appetite isn't so good and why I feel fatigued much of the time. She says it's also why my resistance to colds is so low and my blood pressure is too high. She tells me that I don't do myself any good by getting angry or upset so easily, or by always being in such a rush to get things done. I don't quite get the connection between all these different things. I've read articles about stress, but I don't really know what it is, or what to do about it. The doctor says to relax, but she doesn't say *how*.

We can suggest some techniques for relaxation, but first, let's try to clear up your understanding of stress. Stress is simply the wear and tear on the body caused by the challenges of living. These challenges, also known as *stressors*, are many and varied. They include factors in the physical environment, like pollutants of air or water, radiation, and disease agents. These are challenges that require us to adapt in order to maintain body health. But psychosocial factors can also be stressors, events like getting married, winning the lottery, losing a job, or losing a spouse. The common denominator seems to be a requirement that we adapt, that we cope, that we accommodate to change.

Our perception of that requirement activates a series of biochemical changes that affect many organs of the body, including the heart, lungs, stomach, kidneys, and immune system. Collectively, all these changes are known as the *stress response.*

It sounds very complicated. It also sounds very automatic—like there is nothing one can do about it.

We need not go into the technical details here. Fortunately, the process is *not* completely automatic, like a reflex. In order for the stimulus—the stressor—to activate the stress response, a number of immediate steps have to occur. If it is a psychosocial stressor, we first have to recognize the event and perceive it as a challenge. Then we have to evaluate its *salience*, its relevance to ourselves and the degree to which it poses a threat to our physical or psychological well-being. If we ignore a stimulus, or view it as unimportant, then it won't trigger a stress response. Finally, we have to evaluate our available coping resources and decide how well they can meet the challenge. The most intense and prolonged stress responses appear to get activated when we view ourselves as unable to meet a challenge we evaluate as highly threatening.

I always thought stress was bad for you and should be avoided at all costs. But you say it can occur in so many different kinds of situations. It almost sounds like stress is part of life.

That is quite true. Stress is not the same as distress. The process of adaptation goes on as long as we are living, so stress is, indeed, a part of life. We cannot avoid it altogether, but we can learn to manage it better and to reduce its harmful effects.

If the stress response is supposed to help us adapt, how can it have harmful effects?

That's a very good question. It turns out that some of the chemical changes that are useful in the short run can be harmful if prolonged. One example is the chemical *adrenaline*, which increases its activity as part of the stress response. It elevates blood pressure, which can be helpful in certain acute emergencies, such as those requiring strength or speed, but over the long haul such an effect can be harmful. Other components of the stress reponse increase muscle tension. This, too, is useful when strength and speed are adaptive, for example, when you have to mobilize yourself to run away from an attacker, but over time, tense muscles can lead to headache and chronic low-back or neck pain.

Another response to stress is the increase in chemicals known as *corticosteroids*, which help the blood to clot and are useful in the short run, especially if one is wounded. But they also increase the fatty deposits that clog arteries and can precipitate heart attacks. Still another example is the reduction in activity of our immune systems, which fight disease. All these are aspects of the stress response that can become injurious to health over time.

How can such physical processes be initiated by psychosocial events? You mentioned winning the lottery or losing a spouse. I don't see the connection.

That's because, like most of us, you are accustomed to thinking of the mind and the body as two very different, even opposite, things. We prefer to view them as separate aspects of a single entity—namely, a living organism. Think of the two faces of a coin. Are the "heads" and "tails" two different things, or components of a single thing? If you subjected the coin to a severe environmental challenge, like extreme heat or crushing force, it is unlikely that only one face would be affected, leaving the other unchanged. Mind and body share the same sort of unity. It doesn't matter whether the stressor you are facing threatens your physical or emotional well-being—the body responds in the same way.

Can you give me an example of how that works in my case?

Certainly. We know that some environments are more stressful than others. A country devastated by war or natural disaster, for example, contains more potential stressors than a prosperous nation at peace. Your current environment—that of a primary AD caregiver—is highly stressful. You are continually being challenged by events that tax your available coping resources. You, like all of us, were born with a genetic inheritance that limits the body's ability to adapt. You can think of it as a kind of trust fund, if you will, deposited in your name. Your personal stress trust fund is the total amount of stress that your body will be able to tolerate in your lifetime. It is finite, and it can be wasted. You can choose how and when to make withdrawals from your "stress account," but you can't make any deposits. You can use it up, but you can't replenish it.

The size and nature of the account varies from one person to another, so some people are more susceptible to the adverse effects of stress. Their genetic endowment may leave them with severely limited adaptive capacity, or with one or more "weak links" in the body systems. At present, there isn't anything we can do to change the genetic blueprint, but there is much we can do within our own lifestyles to reduce the stressful effects of environmental challenges.

Do you mean that I can learn to spend my adaptive resources wisely and not go running to my stress account too often or too long?

Precisely.

I'd certainly like to hear how this is done, especially since my life contains so many stressors right now.

This is all the more reason for you to intervene, so that your stress response does not get activated too often or stay activated for too long.

Intervene? I don't get it.

Remember what we said about psychosocial stressors—the kind you are facing now. These are stimuli, but they don't automatically produce a prolonged stress response unless you evaluate them and *dwell* on them as highly threatening and beyond your ability to cope.

That *is* the way I feel sometimes—taxed beyond my ability.

Feeling helpless is, itself, a potent stressor. Recent evidence suggests that when people see themselves as having no choices, no control over their own lives, they are likely to suffer increased stress along with its adverse effects on health. So, the more you get stuck in self-pity and "poor-me" thinking, and the more you "awfulize" and tell yourself that you cannot stand your difficult and unfortunate situation, the more you are likely to be plagued with fatigue, high blood pressure, and low resistance to disease.

Does it really boil down to what I tell myself? I mean, can I magically change a stressor to a nonstressor just by changing my self-talk?

No. There is no magic, nor is stress management as black and white as that. Frank will, in all likelihood, continue to interrupt your sleep with his nighttime wanderings, and lack of rest is stressful. He will continue to require constant supervision, taking time away from other responsibilities you have, including the responsibility to take care of yourself. This, too, is stressful. You can't *make* him sleep through the night and you can't *make* him self-sufficient. But you don't have to add anger, helplessness, and guilt to the package. You can develop greater patience and greater tolerance for frustration, and you can slow down your hectic pace. You can learn not to get angry or upset so often. You can seek and find options and choices, albeit not great ones.

My doctor mentioned some of these things, too—rushing around frantically, impatient and irritable all the time, getting angry—do these activate the stress response?

Indeed they do. They are aspects of what has been

referred to as "Type A" behavior, a pattern associated with increased risk of developing coronary heart disease.

I thought only high-powered executives with million-dollar budgets had these problems.

That is far from true, and people caring for AD victims can easily fall into Type A or other maladaptive behavior patterns. In fact, *any* of the dysfunctional emotional and behavioral patterns we've discussed throughout these conversations with caregivers can adversely affect health by activating and prolonging the stress response: anger, perfectionism, guilt, being all things to all people, needing approval, self-pity, self-downing and depression, helplessness, passivity, and nonassertiveness. All these stem from dysfunctional thought, attitudes, and beliefs, and all can be changed. By working diligently to alter your self-talk, you will actually be reducing stress—not by eliminating stressors that are beyond your power to change, but by reevaluating their threat to you and your own ability to cope. These are known as cognitive methods of stress management.

I think I'm beginning to understand. Frank will continue to wander, to behave inappropriately, and to interrupt me with the same questions over and over again. But I don't have to view these things as intolerable, I don't have to insist that he stop acting dementedly, and I don't have to demand of myself that I continue to do all that I used to do in exactly the same ways—and get overwhelmed.

You *are* beginning to understand. How do you expect you will feel when you make these cognitive changes?

Far less angry and far less upset. If I follow you correctly, this emotional change will, in itself, tend to reduce the negative effects of stress on me. Not to mention the benefits of some behavioral changes I could make, such as managing my time better by setting priorities and doing the most important things and letting the rest wait till another day. After all, where is it written that my carpets must be vacuumed and my floors scrubbed daily?

Where, indeed?

That idea will be hard for me to let go, though, because I've always prided myself on my ability to manage my household affairs well. Now I'll have to face the fact that I can't do it as well as I used to. I'm afraid that doesn't leave me feeling very good about myself.

Don't forget that you have assumed a second, and even more challenging, set of responsibilities in addition to those of running your home. You are now the principal caregiver of a demented adult. It is quite unrealistic to expect that this second job won't impede your performance in the first.

Even more importantly, aren't you equating your skill as a homemaker with your worth as a human being? Does that seem logical to you?

That *is* what I'm doing—and what I've long been doing, I suspect. No, it doesn't seem logical. Does this sort of thinking also produce stress?

Sure. What could be more stressful than putting yourself down as ineffectual and worthless? How well can such a person be expected to cope with the challenges of life?

Not very well. So, if I put myself down, then every potential stressor seems even more threatening, while I seem inadequate to cope.

And that adds up to more intense and persistent stress, with more adverse effects on health.

O.K. So the more realistically I can view myself, Frank, and his illness, the less stress. Is there anything else I can do?

Yes. We referred earlier to relaxation methods of stress management. These include a variety of techniques for "tuning down" those body systems activated as part of the stress response. Deep, slow, diaphragmatic breathing is one of these techniques; muscle relaxation is another; imagery, self-hypnosis, and meditation are still others. A suggested relaxation exercise is outlined in Chapter Fourteen, and you will find references to books and audio-cassettes in the References section.

Finally, you can put into practice the principles of a sound lifestyle: exercise, good nutrition, adequate rest (which in your case may require you to seek respite care for Frank), limited use of alcohol, therapeutic use only of other drugs, and abstinence from smoking.

PART **III**

What Is, *Is:*
Acceptance

CHAPTER **12**

What I Can and Cannot Change

You have gone through the process of dismay, disbelief, and denial until you finally faced the reality of your relative's Alzheimer's disease. Acceptance of this harsh reality has been difficult, but you learned that denial can only lead to maladaptive behavior, while acceptance of reality leads to successful coping in a situation that is at best, sad, and at worst, tragic.

Does acceptance mean passivity and hopelessness? No, indeed. It means changing what you can change and accepting what you cannot.

Realistic acceptance of your situation involves a four-fold process:

1. Acceptance of the fact that you can change how you feel

In the previous chapters, we saw how to apply the principles of RET, or cognitive restructuring, to the gamut of emotions that you, like most caregivers, experience.

We have compartmentalized these emotions as if

each was called forth at a given moment as a separate and distinct feeling. Although this is not entirely accurate, we have done so in order to clarify the nature of emotional responses and their relationship to your perceptions of events. Emotional responses are generally overlapping and complex. You may simultaneously feel rage, self-pity and shame. By identifying your feelings and relating them to your misperceptions and overgeneralizations you can learn to change those which prevent you from making the best possible decisions for yourself and for your loved one.

Along the way, many of you have undoubtedly said, "Yes, but . . ." We understand you mean, "Yes, I understand what you are saying, but it doesn't work. What you are saying makes sense intellectually, but I still feel furious, I still feel pretty sorry for myself, and I still feel guilty."

Intellectual acceptance of the basic premises of RET is the first step in the process of emotional change. But intellectual acceptance does not bring about emotional change. Learning to change your thoughts is the second step. Incorporating the new, more adaptive thoughts into your everyday life is the third step. This is a process that takes daily awareness, daily applications, and daily practice. Emotional change and behavioral change then follow.

In the first century A.D., Epictetus, the Greek philosopher, said, "Men [and we add women] are disturbed, not by events, but by the views they take of them." In *Hamlet,* Shakespeare expressed a similar thought: "There is nothing good or bad, but thinking makes it so."

Neither of these statements implies that your loved one's illness is a figment of your imagination, or that it is a neutral or indifferent event. It does mean that your perception of the event is what you bring to the objective situation. The objective situation is the chronic, deteriorative illness of your family member, with all that implies of changed relationships, dashed hopes, failed expectations, and pain.

You can't change your objective reality. Acceptance means acknowledgment of what *is*, no matter how unfair, unfortunate, or unpleasant. It means taking reality as a given and doing the best you can within the limits of the possible.

What you can change is your "thinking makes it so"—your evaluation of the situation, how you define it. You have learned how to change your thinking, by substituting realistic self-statements for "awfulizing," self-destructive ones.

Emotional change does not rob you of your emotional range. It does not make an unfeeling automaton of you. That would not be possible nor desirable. It does help you to damp down rage; to give up self-pity; to substitute the possible for guilt-producing perfectionism; to reduce anxiety to a manageable level; to feel sadness without sliding into depression; to accept your human fallibility.

2. Acceptance of the disease process and its downhill course over an indeterminate period of time

You have been helped by the fact that Alzheimer's disease is now out of the closet; that it is a disease, worthy of a name other than "senility"; that it is a disease primarily of the latter part of life, just as measles is a disease primarily of the early years, but is no more an inevitable stage of aging than measles is an inevitable illness of the young. You are buoyed by the knowledge that it is now a subject of serious

research and the hope that someday science will dis-
cover a preventive as effective for AD as a vaccine
is for measles.

You have learned to reject time-honored stereotypes
and to look critically at the latest "breakthrough."
And, while you don't give up hope that some way
will be found to ease your loved one's condition, you
don't succumb to the false hope of a "cure" that will
reverse your relative's condition.

3. Acceptance of the patient and her full humanity

Acceptance means accepting your loved one, not as
the person she was, but as the person she is becoming.
That means accepting her in her totality, with all of
her deficits, dementia, difficulties, and demands. It
means acknowledging that profound changes are taking place in her brain and that these changes cause
her to behave in strange ways.

Your afflicted relative is in the process of losing her
ability to reason, to remember, to make sense out of
her world, and to relate to the people in it. She doesn't
lose these abilities at once, nor does she lose them at
a uniform rate. That is why her behavior seems so
in-and-out; why she carries on a lucid conversation
some times, and at other times doesn't know who you
are, or where she is.

While losing her cognitive abilities, she still main-
tains the ability to feel. She has emotions—sometimes
blunted, sometimes exaggerated. But she can still feel
anger, pain, sorrow, hurt, gladness, and pleasure. She
can still respond to affection, to approval, to an acknowledgment that she is a worthwhile person. She
is struggling for affirmation of her humanity.

Accepting her with all the deficits that Alzheimer's

inflicts helps you to reach out to her and to communicate to her your understanding that she is no less
human than before. And human beings deserve respect.

4. Acceptance of the effect your loved one's illness is having on your life

Whatever your previous relationship to your parent,
your spouse, or your elderly uncle, you are now the
caregiver, and he is your dependent. This is a profound
change that you hardly anticipated. Whatever you
had hoped to do at this time of your life, the central
fact is your responsibility for your sick family member. Perhaps you had hoped that in your middle years
you would reap the benefit of having raised your
children; of having struggled through the early years
of financial difficulty to relative financial security; of
having weathered the rough spots in your own marriage. Perhaps you have embarked on a new, more
satisfying marriage, or are experiencing for the first
time the freedom of being single. Or were hoping that
your mate would begin to look after you now that
you were beginning to experience the aches and pains
of your own old age.

You now find yourself the primary—or sole—caregiver of a deteriorating, dementing patient.

You are faced with having to make many decisions,
the most difficult being how much of your own, or
your family's, life you are willing and able to commit
to the sick person's care.

Acceptance of your situation means recognizing:

• Your own limitations as a caregiver
• Your human need for help
• Your human right to ask for that help

If you are asking whether acceptance will banish all emotional pain and turmoil, the answer is *no.* Acceptance facilitates coping. It does not guarantee mastery.

And acceptance of your situation means seeking and finding better options to deal with a difficult reality. It means seizing the initiative and creating opportunities to improve a tough situation wherever possible. It means saying to yourself, "This is what I have; how can I make it just a little bit better?"

CHAPTER **13**

Dealing with Strange or Unexpected Behaviors

You have just examined your emotional responses to your relative's deteriorating state. You have seen how you can apply the principles of Rational Emotive Therapy to reduce your more extreme emotional responses to manageable levels. You have learned that emotions don't just come out of your gut or your heart, but that your gut and your heart respond to what's in your head. And that what is in your head is largely under your control. You can change what is in your head. That is what is called *cognitive restructuring*, which simply means that by examining your evaluations of what is happening, and changing them to more reasonable and realistic evaluations, your emotions become less extreme and therefore more adaptable. This requires a good deal of effort on your part. But you will find yourself well rewarded for the effort.

Without the added burden of extreme stress, rage, anxiety, guilt, or depression, you can develop more flexible coping skills that will improve the care you give your loved one and open new possibilities for your own life.

The fastidious husband refuses to bathe; the loving father doesn't know you; the old friend orders you out of her house; the gentle wife has become a suspicious shrew; your garrulous sister has become withdrawn and mute; the autocratic family head has become a frightened dove. In the face of disorganized behavior, your established repertory of responses no longer serves you. You feel at a loss for appropriate responses.

In this chapter, we will examine some of the more common behaviors that AD patients manifest from time to time, and we will give you some suggestions for handling them.

Not everyone is alike. These suggestions may work with some patients and not others; they may work sometimes, but not every time; they may not work at all. The important message is that caring for an AD patient can be a challenge to your ability to be flexible and creative in the face of unfamiliar, obnoxious, or even dangerous behaviors.

Before we present specifics, we would like to discuss some general principles to serve as guidelines and to dispel some myths about AD patients.

SOME COMMON MYTHS

To understand your patient better, it's wise to give up the idea that AD—or any form of senile dementia—is analogous to second childhood. This erroneous notion has become embedded in popular wisdom and is often perpetuated by writers on the subject. But if you think of your relative in terms of childhood behaviors, you will be very wide of the mark. The only thing your patient and a child have in common is dependency due to an inability to take care of himself. A child is eager, inquisitive, constantly adding new information and processing it to form stable images of the world and his place in it. The AD patient is grappling with the loss of a lifetime of once-learned, once-stable images. He can no longer process new information. With increasing memory and cognitive loss, his store of information is slowly eroded. With loss of language skills, his conceptual processes diminish. This loss of mental abilities threatens his very sense of self.

A child's horizons are constantly expanding. The AD patient's horizons are diminishing. That is why your relative clings to sameness, familiarity, fewer stimuli. Even the familiar becomes unfamiliar, as his brain deteriorates and old knowledge is lost.

AD is a disease process. It is erroneous to view a disease process as analogous to a normal developmental stage, even in reverse.

Because of the constriction of mental abilities, a condition called *concreteness* sets in. That is, the patient can only deal with very specific objects or situations, not with ideas. For example, he may not be able to answer the question, "What would you like to do today?" He would more likely respond to, "Would you like to take a walk," or better still, "Let's take a walk."

Attempts at logical discussion are futile. He can no longer follow a logical sequence. Therefore, any attempt to explain logically that you didn't steal his watch can only meet with great resistance. There are better ways of handling such accusations, as we will see later on.

Another fallacy of popular wisdom is that people just naturally become stubborn when they get old, and you'd better not let them get away with it. This idea often leads to destructive clashes of will. What appears to be stubbornness is generally defensive behavior on the part of the brain-impaired person. His so-called stubbornness may be his way of trying to preserve his personal integrity in the face of a world he can no longer comprehend.

There are many components to what appears to be a simple response to a simple request. But even the simplest human behavior is not simple. For example: If you say to your relative, "Now, go into the bathroom and brush your hair," you may be quite upset if he wanders in the opposite direction. But look at the sequence of events that must be activated between your request and an appropriate response:

1. *Attention:* Your relative must *select* your request out of the welter of stimuli impinging upon him at that moment and *focus* his attention upon your words
2. *Information processing:* Your relative must maintain the focus of his attention long enough for your words to be *processed* by his brain
3. *Comprehension:* His brain must be able to convert those verbal stimuli into a form from which it can extract the *meaning* of your words, thus making comprehension of your request possible
4. *Memory:* Your relative must be able to *retain* the information contained in your request long enough to act upon it
5. *Planning a response:* Your relative must be able to exercise sufficient *judgment* to decide upon an appropriate strategy for dealing with your request, which

includes the appropriate *sequencing* of several separate actions—*recalling* where the bathroom is; knowing how to get there; *identifying* the proper tool for brushing one's hair and how to *use* it; and recognizing when the sequence is finished and being able to *terminate* it

6. *Execution:* Your relative's brain must be able to issue the mental commands to appropriate muscles of the body in order to *execute* the response

Only then can the appropriate response occur. Disruption of any part of this sequence results in failure to respond appropriately. Your brain-impaired relative may be impaired in any or all of these processes. Memory is one link in the sequence, and memory loss is the most recognizable.

Memory loss is part of the problem. It can also be an ally to you, the caregiver, in the daily management of the patient. It enables you to use diversion as a constructive alternative to clashes of will when your patient refuses to do something you think is important, such as taking pills, or insists on doing something you think is inappropriate, such as going out of doors in his underwear. Collisions, or clashes of will, are usually counterproductive and frequently precipitate catastrophic reactions. Such clashes arouse the suspicions in your patient that you do not trust him, do not respect his integrity as a person, and are denying him the right to make decisions for himself. Creatively using memory loss to bring about more amenable behavior is generally the more fruitful alternative.

Another fallacy of popular wisdom is that the obnoxious traits, such as paranoia, that have begun to manifest themselves in the diseased person were there all along but submerged, and that for some reason they are now surfacing in an exaggerated form. There is no evidence for such a view.

Personality is an expression of genetic predisposi- ton, environment, socialization processes, acting on a substrate of a given brain and body. As the brain deteriorates, altered processes are generated. These processes may have little or no continuity with the lifelong personality and behavior of your relative. Old ways of responding, based on an intact brain, are disrupted. New ones, responding to the messages em- anating from the damaged brain, erupt. The new be- haviors are chaotic and generally incomprehensible.

However, some aspects of your relative's behavior often remain intact, at least for a long time. The sick individual continues to want reassurance and affec- tion, especially from those closest to him. He is often aware of his deficits—his inability to find words, his difficulty in controlling bodily functions, how hard it is to make himself understood. When he finds himself unable to manage everyday communication and or- dinary controls, long taken for granted, he often feels intensely frustrated and humiliated. He is grateful for your assurances that he is O.K., that you understand, that you don't judge him, and that you love him.

WHAT TO DO OR SAY AT DIFFICULT MOMENTS

On the theory that forthrightness and total honesty can sometimes be the worst policy, we use creative evasions; half-truths that give comfort; reassurance instead of criticism; diversion instead of clashes of will. Instead of logic, we find ways of empathically putting ourselves into the patient's frame of reference.

———•◆•———

Your mother has just accused you of having stolen

her new blouse. You become very hurt that she could believe that of you. You explain, patiently, that (1) you just bought it for her; (2) her blouse would not fit you; (3) you don't want it; and (4) you are not a thief, you have never been a thief, and you resent the accusation, especially in view of all you are doing for her. Your mother becomes enraged, and you break down in tears.

Instead of letting yourself be hurt by your mother's accusation, ignore the provocation. Tell her, "Let's look in your closet together. We'll probably find it." When you find it—as you probably will—say, "Isn't it lucky that we found your blouse?" If you haven't found it (she may have hidden it someplace), you might try, "We'll look for it again after we've had our lunch." A scene has been averted. She'll appreciate a hug.

———•———

Your wife turns to you one day and says, "Who are you?" You feel devastated. You become angry and say, "You know perfectly well who I am." Or, "Stop playing games with me." Or you make a disparaging remark— "Are you out of your mind?" She feels hurt and more confused. You feel hurt, bewildered, and frightened.

A better reaction would be simply to answer, in a reassuring manner, "I am Burt, your husband. I live here with you." Repeat this as often as necessary. If it becomes more repetitive than you can reasonably put up with, divert her: "Look at this snapshot of our grandchild, Emily. Isn't she cute?" Or, "It's television time now." And lead her by the hand to the TV.

———•———

Your husband is cowering in the bedroom and refuses to come out. He says that "they" are out there.

"They" are a group of men in dark clothing who are out to get him. You explain that there's no one out there. You open the door and turn on the light. You show him that there's no one there. But he knows better, because he sees them, and maybe you think he's crazy, but he knows he isn't. He becomes agitated.

Instead of using logic, and the rules of evidence, try the following: "Hold my hand, and together we'll chase them away. Let's call out first and tell them we're coming. That will scare them." Take your husband's hand firmly, shout at "them" and then, with some gusto, open the door. "See, they're gone. There's no one here." This engages your husband in his own security and gives him a sense of mastery over the frightful, and frightening, apparitions that his mind conjures up. You might also suggest, "If they ever come back again, just let me know, and we'll get rid of them again." He knows that he can depend on you.

By acting empathically, from the point of view of his frame of reference, you neither confirm nor reinforce his delusion. You do not suggest that you, too, see "them." You are showing him that (1) he doesn't have to be afraid of "them"; and (2) you are willing to help him. You establish trust.

———•———

Your father refuses to go to bed. He remains in the bathroom, clutching his toothbrush, his hairbrush, and his shaving cream. You are nonplussed. You try to take these objects away from him. He holds on more firmly than ever. You ask him why he won't let go, and he tells you that as soon as he goes to bed, "They'll come and steal them." You tell him, "That's ridiculous. Who would want them?" He refuses to budge. You insist that he go to bed. It's getting late. But he is prepared to stay up all night to defend his possessions. A head-on collision is in the making.

Bring in a brown paper bag and a rubber band or piece of string. Suggest to him, "Let's put these things in the bag and tie it up real tight. Now take it into bed with you. Your things will be perfectly safe that way." Reassured, he does just that. When he falls asleep, put the objects back where they belong. He'll never remember the incident. And he went to bed feeling that his integrity had been respected.

———•———

She is trying to tell you something but can't find the words. She hesitates, and meaningless sounds erupt. She looks humiliated, embarrassed. You stand by, waiting expectantly. You say, "I can't understand a word you're saying. Just try a little harder to get it straight." She becomes more confused. You become impatient, and obviously annoyed. You say, "Never mind." She senses your annoyance, and becomes either angry or withdrawn.

You might guess at what she wants and offer some suggestions. If one proves correct, you might say, "That's fine. I know that's just what you wanted to tell me." If you can't guess, and your relative can't show you what it is that she wants, then it could be helpful, along with a comforting stroke of the hand, to say, "That's O.K., you'll think of it later." Later, she won't remember the episode. Or, "I want to hear what you have to say, but first let's have these nice grapes I bought." Diversion is an excellent antidote to frustration in the AD patient.

———•———

She's decided to report you to the police—for whatever reason. She is furious about some injustice done her. You become indignant and shout at her that she'd better not dare. You grab the phone from her hand. She shouts obscenities. A catastrophic episode follows. You finally have to sedate her.

Instead, quietly say, "Here is the phone. I'm sure the police will be very helpful." She tries to call but can't manage it. You offer to help. You dial some numbers, and then announce, "Sorry we have a busy signal. We'll try again later." "Later" is often a magic word for people with short memories. Then add, "In the meantime, let's play your favorite music on the stereo."

He says, "I haven't seen my mother lately. When is she coming?" You explain that his mother died fifteen years ago. He breaks down and cries bitterly. He asks, "Why didn't anyone tell me?" You remind him that he went to the funeral, and that Aunt Rosalyn and Uncle Harry were there, and all the children and cousins came. He searches his mind, and then says, "I haven't seen my mother lately. When is she coming?"

You realize that explanations are useless, and that in his present fragile state, the truth of his mother's death is too traumatic for him to accept. So, you simply say, "I haven't seen her either in a long time. I'm sure you miss her. So do I. We all miss her. It would certainly be nice to see her again." You have shown him that you understand.

She announces, "I'm going home." She has lived here for thirty years. You explain that this is her home. That she has no other. But she doesn't believe you. She may be dredging up the long-forgotten memory of a childhood home that, to her, is her real home, and she means to go there. You try to convince her that this is her home. She opens the front door and tries to step out into the cold night. A struggle ensues.

You might say, "I understand, but I'd love to have you stay for dinner. We have such a good dinner tonight, and I've been counting on you to stay." The chances are that she'll be happy to accept your invitation. If it's not dinner time, you might suggest having a nice snack together before she leaves. This tells her that she is wanted here but is free to go. It's most likely that she will choose to stay.

"Why don't we ever see Marsha? It's been ages since she was here!" You explain that Marsha—your daughter—has just left. He says that she hasn't been here in four years. You repeat what you just said, that Marsha just left. He looks very dejected. "Are you telling me that I don't know what I'm talking about?" He feels hurt and misunderstood.

Instead, simply say, "Let's call her and tell her we'd love to see her again." We'll call her. He has forgotten what it is he wanted to say. But he feels comforted.

He refuses to bathe, wash, brush his teeth, or shave. You explain that (1) personal hygiene is essential for health; (2) he looks awful, unshaven, unkempt, and ungroomed; and (3) he stinks. You insist that he get into the bath immediately. He refuses. You are beside yourself. You can't put him into the tub—he's too heavy for you. You shout, you cajole, you threaten. He is adamant.

Try a gentler approach. Sweet reason is of no avail to a person who has lost the ability to reason. A clash of will is even more threatening than the bath. So, it's wise to back off and simply say, "That's O.K., you can get washed another time." Later, or the next day, you might say, "Here's your bath, I'll help you in." Or, "You look so comfortable in bed this morning. So here's a nice basin of soapy water. I'm going to give you a sponge bath right here in bed." If neither of these strategies works, you will have to devise your own. But always avoid saying, "You must." Accept his refusal as natural, and try again.

———•—•———

She breaks down and cries for no apparent reason. You feel deeply for her. You are sympathetic. You say, "What's the matter, dear? Why are you crying?" She can't explain to you. She doesn't find words. She becomes more frustrated and more depressed. You feel helpless—it's no use, because you really tried.

Better still, when you see her crying, touch her, stroke her hand, put your arms around her, and say, "I know that you feel frustrated and sad. Things are getting hard for you. But I'm here to help." Then you might try diverting her with a suggestion like, "Come help me fix dinner." This makes her feel loved, understood, and useful.

———•—•———

It's evening. Almost bedtime. That's generally the hardest time of day. Suddenly he says, "Where am I?" He looks around the room. "I don't know where I am. I don't know who I am." He looks terrified. To lose contact with one's environment, and with one's sense of self, is to face dissolution of one's self.

You don't know what to do to help. You say, "You are overtired. I'll help you to bed." He can't comprehend your words. You, too, are frightened.

Instead, touching him lightly, quietly say, "You are Steve Gold. I am your wife, Ann Gold. This is your home. You are in the living room. You are in the living room of your home. This is your easy chair. Let's touch it. Let's walk around and look at everything. This is the armchair, and this is the coffee table. Let's touch them.''

Repeat this, quietly walking around the house, identifying each room, naming objects, touching them as you name them, repeating his name and yours.

Eventually, he will reorient himself. His environment will again come into focus. His sense of his own identity will return.

———•———

He sits and stares blankly. Then he says, "I want to die." That is frightening. You don't know what to say. Part of you tells yourself, "I don't blame him. I would want to die, too, if I were in his condition." Then you feel guilty and say to yourself, "That's not right. Life is a precious gift. We just don't give up, no matter what." So you say nothing, and hope that he doesn't mention it again. He may think that you are indifferent to his pain and indeed may not mention it again.

It would be better to touch him. Caress him. Tell him that you don't want him to die, that you would miss him if he were gone. Tell him that you understand that life is very hard for him and that you understand his frustration. Tell him that Marion and Richard, the children, love him and want him to be here a long time. And then do something that he previously enjoyed, like listening to music, reading a few pages from a favorite book, taking a walk, or watching TV. This helps to reaffirm a sense of commitment to life.

———•———

We have just presented some examples that demonstrate what we consider to be appropriate and generally successful methods of dealing with some of the more difficult moments in the family caregiver–AD patient relationship.

These fragments don't presume to cover all possible difficulties. And they are not offered as a catalogue of surefire cookbook recipes for handling Alzheimer's patients.

However, they do represent a point of view based on the following principles:

1. Avoid head-on collisions whenever possible.
2. Make use of the patient's memory loss to divert and rechannel asocial, obnoxious, or potentially destructive behavior.
3. Give reassurance, affection, and emotional support.
4. Show respect for his integrity by acting as if his perceptions—no matter how distorted—are valid. This establishes trust and enables you to deal with his misperceptions in a constructive way.
5. Be creative.

Coping with an Alzheimer's relative can be a painful challenge. But remember: In spite of your best efforts, you can't solve all the problems.

CHAPTER **14**

Be Good to Yourself

You are now going through the painful process of reorienting your life in ways that you never anticipated. Events have forced new meanings to the commandment that you learned and accepted as a child: "Honor thy father and thy mother." Your marriage vow, which joined you "in sickness and in health till death do us part," has assumed a reality of which you were hardly aware in the youthful days of optimism and promise. And your value system of care and concern for suffering humanity is being tested in an arena far from the faceless tragedies of famine and drought and earthquakes. It has been transported into your own home, to your own relative, your own loved one.

You have sought help from doctors, some whose ignorance was matched only by lack of concern; some who cared but were helpless to guide you; some who saw the patient as a "case" to be studied, and you as someone to be ignored; some who mollified you by giving you worthless prescriptions and false hopes;

and some—a growing body within the medical profession—who were actively seeking knowledge in what looked like an epidemic of growing proportions, and who showed an increased awareness that Alzheimer's is a disease affecting not only the patient, but the entire family, with you, the caregiver, at the core.

You get overwhelmed by advice, good, bad, and contradictory. And the bottom line, for you, is: How do you solve the human equation between your patient's needs and your own? Just as nothing about AD is easy, the answer to that question is not easy. So much depends on your own physical, emotional, financial, and social resources. That being the case, you have to solve the equation yourself. But never forget that you are part of the equation.

In this book, we have shown you how to deal constructively with the emotional responses of living with, and caring for, a person who is slowly changing from an integrated human being capable of functioning in the world to a dependent, demented adult. At the same time that you are learning the cognitive restructuring that brings about emotional change, there are some practical steps that you can take to help you to reorder your life.

ENDING ISOLATION

Mates of AD patients often call themselves "married widows and widowers." This neatly expresses the social limbo in which they often find themselves. Ending your isolation is your number-one priority. Here are some suggestions:

1. The Alzheimer's Disease and Related Disorders Asso-

ciation (ADRDA) offers you the opportunity to meet other people with similar problems. Local chapters, formed all over the country, provide mutual support, exchange of information, a place for sharing some of your own problems, a chance to learn from others in the same situation, and the opportunity to share with others what you have learned.

To find out about a chapter near you, contact the National Headquarters of ADRDA at:

National ADRDA Office
70 East Lake Street
Chicago, IL 60601
1-800-621-0379

2. Call a family meeting. Very often, the caregiver struggles against great odds to provide total care for the patient, with no assistance of any kind from anyone. The rationales for this range from "It's my job," to "No one else will do it as well," to "I can't impose on anyone else," to "What's the use asking, no one will help anyway." Since care for an AD patient can easily become a twenty-four-hour job, this attitude can lead to physical or emotional breakdown of the caregiver. Neither the caregiver nor the patient is served.

Calling a family meeting (with family defined as broadly as possible to include close family friends and neighbors) serves to acquaint a circle of people with the problem and to elicit some offers of help, however minimally individuals become involved. If you cannot handle such a meeting on your own, perhaps you can get the help of an outsider—a counselor, a church leader, or an experienced member of your ARDRA group. Even if help means relieving you for an occasional evening or afternoon, this opens the way for you to begin to indulge some of your own needs and interests.

3. Look into respite-care and day-care facilities in your

community. Where such facilities exist, they will not only provide you with time off, but will provide an optimum environment for your AD relative.

4. If at all financially possible, try to arrange for part-time paid assistance: one afternoon a week, one evening a week, an occasional weekend—or more if you can afford it.

5. Join an organization that interests you: a church group, social-service group, fund-raising group, discussion group, library book club. You might volunteer to stuff envelopes at home for your favorite charity, or make calls for your favorite political organization. This type of activity can provide links to the broader community while you are confined to your home.

6. Make a list of people you haven't seen for a while. Some old friends may have fallen away because of their own difficulties in dealing with your AD relative. Some may be responding to your withdrawal from social life. Others may be involved in their own problems. You will never know who your viable friends are until you take the initiative to find out. Try calling and suggesting a simple social evening or afternoon. You may have more friends than you think. Or fewer. You may find a whole new resource for new friendships in the support-group meetings that you will now attend.

BE GOOD TO YOURSELF

1. Take care of your own physical health. This involves checkups, proper nutrition, exercise and rest.

   If your patient keeps you awake night after night, try to get someone to cover for you occasionally so that you can get an unbroken night's sleep.

2. Make a list of all the things you enjoy doing, and arrange them in order of priorities. Decide which are most feasible and then make plans for carrying them

out. You might decide that this is the time to go square dancing, or to take that painting class or creative writing class at your local high school adult-education program. Or go bowling or swimming. Indulge your fancy.

3. Make a list of gifts you would like to receive. Not impossible gifts, or wildly extravagant ones fit for a movie star, but ones that are realistic for your budget, ones that you would love to have, but can do without because there's always something more important or more sensible. Give yourself an occasional gift.

LEARN TO RELAX

As we discussed earlier, mind and body are one. Mental tension has its counterpart in physical tension. Strong negative emotions arouse strong physiologic responses and excessive muscular tension. And sustained excessive muscular tension results in wear and tear of your body.

You have at your command a powerful tool to help you defuse the tension that your body builds up in response to the emotional turmoil caused by anger, anxiety, and frustration.

That tool is learning to relax.

We all know the benefits of relaxation. We go to the beach or to the mountains, or take a Caribbean vacation. We say, "When I sit and look at the waves breaking on the rocks, I haven't a care in the world." That's true, because when you sit and look at the waves breaking on the rocks, you allow your muscles to relax. And when your muscles relax, your mind relaxes. You can't feel tense, anxious, and relaxed at the same time.

You can achieve the same state of relaxation in your

own home by *learning* to relax. It takes a little practice—about ten minutes a day at first. Once you have mastered the technique, you will find that you have fewer headaches, fewer backaches, and experience less fatigue.

Here is a relaxation exercise that has proved valuable in many settings:

Begin by getting as comfortable as you can in a reclining chair, sofa, or bed. Make sure that your head and neck, arms, back, and legs are well-supported. You may wish to remove your shoes and loosen any tight articles of clothing.

Take a deep breath and hold it for a few seconds while you pay attention to the tenseness of your chest muscles. Exhale slowly and notice the same muscles beginning to relax. Repeat this step. You may notice a feeling of calm beginning to develop already.

Now tense all the muscles of your body at once and study how this feels. After counting to five, allow all these muscles to relax—just let all the tension go. Feel yourself sinking into the chair as your muscles let go and you become comfortably heavy, limp, and relaxed. You may be aware of sensations of warmth or tingling as your muscles continue to let go of more and more tension. If your eyes are not already closed, you may allow them to close lightly now.

Starting at the top of your head, scan your body for remaining feelings of muscle tension and passively allow these muscles to relax. Name the parts of your body silently as you proceed slowly, letting go of more and more tension: scalp, forehead, eyes, face, jaws, lips and tongue, throat and neck, shoulders and upper back, arms and fingers, chest, stomach, lower back, hips, thighs, calves, the tips of your toes. Spend about ten minutes enjoying the pleasant sensations of looseness and relaxation as your muscles just let go.

Now, with your eyes closed, imagine you are traveling to a very beautiful and peaceful place. It can be an actual place or one that exists only in fantasy. Use all your senses to create a vivid mental image of this place. See the shapes and colors, hear the sounds, smell the aromas, and feel the textures of this place. Pay attention to how comfortable and relaxed you feel while you are in this place. Cares and concerns, aches and pains, all seem to float far away.

You may return to this place as often as you like and remain as long as you wish, feeling as peaceful and relaxed as you do now. When you are ready to return to the present, simply count from one to five, coming closer and closer and feeling more and more alert with each number. When you reach the number five, you will arrive at the present, and you may open your eyes, feeling alert, relaxed, and ready to resume your daily activities.

After some practice, you learn to tune in to various parts of your body. You can use a cue word, like *relax*. Your body, having been trained, will respond to the cue and, indeed, will relax. This will help you to reduce your tension as you go about your business. Your onerous tasks will become much less onerous.

You may wish to tape record this exercise and play it as a guide while you practice.

IMAGERY

Imagery is the magic carpet that transports us to faraway places; it changes drab reality to sparkling unreality and endows each of us with Aladdin's lamp.

Imagery can also be used not to wish away our

unhappy reality, but to make it more bearable. It can be used not in the service of escape, but in the service of adaptation. Here's how:

Make yourself comfortable. Relax. Now think of a particularly difficult episode relating to your AD patient. For example: You have just gotten her fully dressed and are ready to leave the house together for a doctor's appointment. She suddenly decides to take off her clothes and take a bath. You explain, you cajole. No use.

In imagery—since you are in command—you remain calm. You do not allow yourself to get rattled. You try diversion. At the very worst, you give your patient her bath and start all over again. It's all in a day's work. You calmly call the doctor and make another appointment. Nothing terrible has happened. You have seen yourself through this episode with no emotional storms, either on her part or yours.

But, you say, this was all in my imagination. I can do anything I want in imagination. That's not real life.

No, it isn't real life, but it can be an effective rehearsal for real life, because your body responds to your imaginings in the same way as in real life. So, if you practice, through imagery, remaining calm in the face of what might be severe provocation, you are practicing a skill that will be at your command when real provocations occur.

The more you employ imagery, the more available this calming response will become when the need arises.

COGNITIVE PRACTICE

You are learning to replace maladaptive self-statements, such as "Poor me," "It isn't fair," "It's terrible," "I can't stand it," with more adaptive ones, such as "I don't like it, but I can stand it," "The world is not fair," "It's unfortunate, but not terrible." To help you internalize the more adaptive messages, you might make cue cards with messages written out and place them in strategic places, such as above your bathroom mirror, over the kitchen sink, next to your bed. These serve as reminders that, hard as it is, you can cope. Repeat the messages to yourself, as often as possible.

PREPARE YOURSELF FOR EMERGENCIES

1. In spite of promises you made to yourself, your patient, or your family, there may come a time when it will be necessary to send your loved one to a nursing home. This may be a sudden decision, based upon your inability to continue to give care, or may result from the rapid deterioration of your relative's condition.

   Now is the time to investigate nursing homes and to familiarize yourself with the quality of care and its cost. It is best to be prepared.

2. Acquaint yourself with government agencies in your community that can provide some help. Become familiar with financial arrangements and any sources of financial help that may become necessary.

3. Keep a list of important phone numbers handy: police, ambulance service, doctors.

   Since few private physicians pay house calls any longer, it is wise to locate the services of medical groups that do send out doctors on house calls. Your patient may, at some time, require immediate attention, and he may not be in a position to be taken to your doctor's office or a hospital emergency room.

4. Keep a list of those people whom you can call upon to help out in case of emergency.

5. BE GOOD TO YOURSELF. YOU DESERVE IT.

Epilogue: I'm Only Human

It is now two months since Mike died, I am experiencing a strange reaction from friends and family. They look at me and then in a tone of amazement say, "You look so well, Irene."

I understand why people are so surprised at my appearance. I am supposed to be the bereaved widow. And I'm not.

Why aren't you? Didn't you love Mike?

Yes, I loved Mike very much. But the Mike I loved left me many years ago. I mourned his passing for six long years, as his mind slowly slipped away. When finally his body followed, my mourning was almost completed.

How could you have mourned a living person whom you saw daily and whom you nurtured?

This was a process that was imperceptible at first. It was a slow process of denial, then acknowledgment; of acceptance, then of emotional disengagement.

I realized that he was no longer a husband, or a lover, or a friend. He was no longer a person with whom I could share my feelings, any experiences, or any decisions. He was no longer a father to our grown children, or a grandfather to the little ones.

Then what was he to you?

He was a dependent. But not just any dependent. He was a dependent whom I loved, even as I was angry with the fate that brought him to this pass. He was a dependent whom I loved, even as I hated his dependency, and, at times, him, for his dependency. He was a dependent whom I loved and mourned, even as I raged inwardly, at times, at what he was doing to my life.

You say you raged inwardly at times. As you learned to apply the principles of Rational Emotive Therapy, or cognitive restructuring, wasn't your rage dispelled?

Yes, in my everyday coping strategies. I learned to say, and to believe, that his bizarre behavior was the result of his deteriorated brain and not the result of an evil disposition or a malignant fate. I learned to ask myself, "How does a demented person behave?" and to answer, "Dementedly." I learned to accept the proposition that the world is not fair, and that there is no rational reason why it should be fair. I learned to stop feeling sorry for myself and to go about the business of living as best I could within the constraints of his illness. I stopped bemoaning our lost dreams of a golden age together.

But deep down, there remained a residue of rage and self-pity. This was an unshakeable bastion of irrationality. I recognized it as such, and I accepted it. This was, and is, part of my human fallibility. As long as I acknowledged it, and understood it, it didn't erupt often, or seriously, into my everyday life. When it did, I didn't allow myself the added burden of guilt for not being perfect. I forgave myself—usually.

When he died, my mourning ended. My rage and my self-pity ended. Only my love for the person who was, and for the unhappy person he became, remained.

References

Brown, D. 1984. *Handle With Care: A Question of Alzheimer's*. Buffalo, NY: Prometheus.

Beck, A. *Rational Thinking: An Antidote to Depression*. Audio-cassette tape #20294, *Psychology Today* Tapes. American Psychological Association, 1200 Seventeenth Street, N.W., Washington, D.C., 20036.

Burns, D. 1980. *Feeling Good*. New York: Signet Books.

Cohen, C. and C. Eisdorfer. 1986. *The Loss of Self*. New York: Norton.

Ellis, A. 1962. *Reason and Emotion in Psychotherapy*. Secaucus, NJ: Citadel Press.

——— 1977. *How to Live With and Without Anger*. New York: Readers Digest Press.

——— and R. Harper 1975. *A New Guide to Rational Living*. North Hollywood, CA: Wilshire Books.

——— and I. Becker. (1982). *A Guide to Personal Hapiness*. North Hollywood, CA: Wilshire Books.

Guthrie, D. 1986. *Grandpa Doesn't Know It's Me*. New York: Human Science Press

Hauck, P. 1973. *Overcoming Depression*. Philadelphia, PA: Westminster Press.

Heston, L. and J. White 1983. *Dementia: A Practical Guide to Alzheimer's Disease and Related Illnesses*. San Francisco, CA: W. H. Freeman.

Jakubowski, P. and A. Lange. 1978. *The Assertive Option*. Champaign, IL: Research Press.

Lazarus, A. *Learning to Relax*. Audio-cassette tape. Institute for Rational Living, 45 East 65th Street, New York.

223

Manning, D. 1986. *The Nursing Home Dilemma: How to Make One of Love's Toughest Decisions.* New York: Harper & Row.

Mace, N. and P. Rabins. 1981. *The 36 Hour Day.* Baltimore: Johns Hopkins University Press.

McDowell, P., ed. 1980. *Managing the Person with Intellectual Loss at Home.* Burke Rehabilitation Center, 785 Mamaroneck Avenue, White Plains, N.Y.

Powell, L. and K. Courtice. 1983. *Alzheimer's Disease: A Guide for Families.* Reading, MA: Addison-Wesley Publishing Co.

Reisberg, B. 1980. *Brain Failure.* New York: The Free Press.

Roach, M. 1985. *Another Name for Madness.* New York: Houghton Mifflin.

Springer, D. and T. Brubecker. 1984. *Family Caregivers and Dependent Elderly.* New York: Sage Publications.

Tanner, F. and S. Shaw. 1985. *Caring: A Family Guide to Managing the Alzheimer's Patient at Home.* New York City Alzheimer's Resource Center, 280 Broadway, New York.

Tavris, C. 1982. *Anger: The Misunderstood Emotion.* New York: Simon & Schuster.

Woolfolk, R. and F. Richardson. 1978. *Stress, Sanity and Survival.* New York: Signet Books.

Zarit, S., N. Orr, and J. Zarit. 1985. *The Hidden Victims of Alzheimer's Disease: Families Under Stress.* New York: New York University Press.

Index

MELVIN POWERS SELF-IMPROVEMENT LIBRARY

COOKERY & HERBS
_____ CULPEPER'S HERBAL REMEDIES *Dr. Nicholas Culpeper*   3.00
_____ FAST GOURMET COOKBOOK *Poppy Cannon*   2.50
_____ GINSENG—THE MYTH & THE TRUTH *Joseph P. Hou*   3.00
_____ HEALING POWER OF HERBS *May Bethel*   4.00
_____ HEALING POWER OF NATURAL FOODS *May Bethel*   5.00
_____ HERBS FOR HEALTH—HOW TO GROW & USE THEM *Louise Evans Doole*   4.00
_____ HOME GARDEN COOKBOOK—DELICIOUS NATURAL FOOD RECIPES *Ken Kraft*   3.00
_____ MEDICAL HERBALIST *Edited by Dr. J. R. Yemm*   3.00
_____ VEGETABLE GARDENING FOR BEGINNERS *Hugh Wiberg*   2.00
_____ VEGETABLES FOR TODAY'S GARDENS *R. Milton Carleton*   2.00
_____ VEGETARIAN COOKERY *Janet Walker*   7.00
_____ VEGETARIAN COOKING MADE EASY & DELECTABLE *Veronica Vezza*   3.00
_____ VEGETARIAN DELIGHTS—A HAPPY COOKBOOK FOR HEALTH *K. R. Mehta*   2.00
_____ VEGETARIAN GOURMET COOKBOOK *Joyce McKinnel*   3.00

HEALTH
_____ BEE POLLEN *Lynda Lyngheim & Jack Scagnetti*   3.00
_____ COPING WITH ALZHEIMER'S *Rose Oliver, Ph.D. & Francis Bock, Ph.D.*   7.00
_____ DR. LINDNER'S SPECIAL WEIGHT CONTROL METHOD *Peter G. Lindner, M.D.*   2.00
_____ HELP YOURSELF TO BETTER SIGHT *Margaret Darst Corbett*   3.00
_____ HOW YOU CAN STOP SMOKING PERMANENTLY *Ernest Caldwell*   5.00
_____ MIND OVER PLATTER *Peter G. Lindner, M.D.*   3.00
_____ NATURE'S WAY TO NUTRITION & VIBRANT HEALTH *Robert J. Scrutton*   3.00
_____ NEW CARBOHYDRATE DIET COUNTER *Patti Lopez-Pereira*   2.00
_____ REFLEXOLOGY *Dr. Maybelle Segal*   4.00
_____ REFLEXOLOGY FOR GOOD HEALTH *Anna Kaye & Don C. Matchan*   5.00
_____ 30 DAYS TO BEAUTIFUL LEGS *Dr. Marc Selner*   3.00
_____ YOU CAN LEARN TO RELAX *Dr. Samuel Gutwirth*   3.00
_____ YOUR ALLERGY—WHAT TO DO ABOUT IT *Allan Knight, M.D.*   3.00

MELVIN POWERS' MAIL ORDER LIBRARY
_____ HOW TO GET RICH IN MAIL ORDER *Melvin Powers*   20.00
_____ HOW TO WRITE A GOOD ADVERTISEMENT *Victor O. Schwab*   20.00
_____ MAIL ORDER MADE EASY *J. Frank Brumbaugh*   20.00

METAPHYSICS & OCCULT
_____ BOOK OF TALISMANS, AMULETS & ZODIACAL GEMS *William Pavitt*   7.00
_____ CONCENTRATION—A GUIDE TO MENTAL MASTERY *Mouni Sadhu*   5.00
_____ EXTRA-TERRESTRIAL INTELLIGENCE—THE FIRST ENCOUNTER   6.00
_____ FORTUNE TELLING WITH CARDS *P. Foli*   5.00
_____ HOW TO INTERPRET DREAMS, OMENS & FORTUNE TELLING SIGNS *Gettings*   5.00
_____ HOW TO UNDERSTAND YOUR DREAMS *Geoffrey A. Dudley*   5.00
_____ IN DAYS OF GREAT PEACE *Mouni Sadhu*   3.00
_____ LSD—THE AGE OF MIND *Bernard Roseman*   2.00
_____ MAGICIAN—HIS TRAINING AND WORK *W. E. Butler*   5.00
_____ MEDITATION *Mouni Sadhu*   7.00
_____ MODERN NUMEROLOGY *Morris C. Goodman*   5.00
_____ NUMEROLOGY—ITS FACTS AND SECRETS *Ariel Yvon Taylor*   5.00
_____ NUMEROLOGY MADE EASY *W. Mykian*   5.00
_____ PALMISTRY MADE EASY *Fred Gettings*   5.00
_____ PALMISTRY MADE PRACTICAL *Elizabeth Daniels Squire*   5.00
_____ PALMISTRY SECRETS REVEALED *Henry Frith*   4.00
_____ PROPHECY IN OUR TIME *Martin Ebon*   2.50
_____ SUPERSTITION—ARE YOU SUPERSTITIOUS? *Eric Maple*   2.00
_____ TAROT *Mouni Sadhu*   10.00
_____ TAROT OF THE BOHEMIANS *Papus*   7.00
_____ WAYS TO SELF-REALIZATION *Mouni Sadhu*   7.00
_____ WITCHCRAFT, MAGIC & OCCULTISM—A FASCINATING HISTORY *W. B. Crow*   7.00
_____ WITCHCRAFT—THE SIXTH SENSE *Justine Glass*   7.00
_____ WORLD OF PSYCHIC RESEARCH *Hereward Carrington*   2.00

SELF-HELP & INSPIRATIONAL

____ CHARISMA—HOW TO GET "THAT SPECIAL MAGIC" *Marcia Grad*	7.00
____ DAILY POWER FOR JOYFUL LIVING *Dr. Donald Curtis*	5.00
____ DYNAMIC THINKING *Melvin Powers*	5.00
____ GREATEST POWER IN THE UNIVERSE *U. S. Andersen*	7.00
____ GROW RICH WHILE YOU SLEEP *Ben Sweetland*	7.00
____ GROWTH THROUGH REASON *Albert Ellis, Ph.D.*	7.00
____ GUIDE TO PERSONAL HAPPINESS *Albert Ellis, Ph.D. & Irving Becker, Ed.D.*	7.00
____ HANDWRITING ANALYSIS MADE EASY *John Marley*	5.00
____ HANDWRITING TELLS *Nadya Olyanova*	7.00
____ HOW TO ATTRACT GOOD LUCK *A.H.Z. Carr*	7.00
____ HOW TO BE GREAT *Dr. Donald Curtis*	5.00
____ HOW TO DEVELOP A WINNING PERSONALITY *Martin Panzer*	5.00
____ HOW TO DEVELOP AN EXCEPTIONAL MEMORY *Young & Gibson*	5.00
____ HOW TO LIVE WITH A NEUROTIC *Albert Ellis, Ph.D.*	7.00
____ HOW TO OVERCOME YOUR FEARS *M. P. Leahy, M.D.*	3.00
____ HOW TO SUCCEED *Brian Adams*	7.00
____ HUMAN PROBLEMS & HOW TO SOLVE THEM *Dr. Donald Curtis*	5.00
____ I CAN *Ben Sweetland*	7.00
____ I WILL *Ben Sweetland*	3.00
____ KNIGHT IN THE RUSTY ARMOR *Robert Fisher*	5.00
____ LEFT-HANDED PEOPLE *Michael Barsley*	5.00
____ MAGIC IN YOUR MIND *U.S. Andersen*	7.00
____ MAGIC OF THINKING BIG *Dr. David J. Schwartz*	3.00
____ MAGIC OF THINKING SUCCESS *Dr. David J. Schwartz*	7.00
____ MAGIC POWER OF YOUR MIND *Walter M. Germain*	7.00
____ MENTAL POWER THROUGH SLEEP SUGGESTION *Melvin Powers*	3.00
____ NEVER UNDERESTIMATE THE SELLING POWER OF A WOMAN *Dottie Walters*	7.00
____ NEW GUIDE TO RATIONAL LIVING *Albert Ellis, Ph.D. & R. Harper, Ph.D.*	7.00
____ PSYCHO-CYBERNETICS *Maxwell Maltz, M.D.*	7.00
____ PSYCHOLOGY OF HANDWRITING *Nadya Olyanova*	7.00
____ SALES CYBERNETICS *Brian Adams*	7.00
____ SCIENCE OF MIND IN DAILY LIVING *Dr. Donald Curtis*	7.00
____ SECRET OF SECRETS *U.S. Andersen*	7.00
____ SECRET POWER OF THE PYRAMIDS *U. S. Andersen*	7.00
____ SELF-THERAPY FOR THE STUTTERER *Malcolm Frazer*	3.00
____ SUCCESS-CYBERNETICS *U. S. Andersen*	7.00
____ 10 DAYS TO A GREAT NEW LIFE *William E. Edwards*	3.00
____ THINK AND GROW RICH *Napoleon Hill*	7.00
____ THINK YOUR WAY TO SUCCESS *Dr. Lew Losoncy*	5.00
____ THREE MAGIC WORDS *U. S. Andersen*	7.00
____ TREASURY OF COMFORT *Edited by Rabbi Sidney Greenberg*	7.00
____ TREASURY OF THE ART OF LIVING *Sidney S. Greenberg*	7.00
____ WHAT YOUR HANDWRITING REVEALS *Albert E. Hughes*	3.00
____ YOUR SUBCONSCIOUS POWER *Charles M. Simmons*	7.00
____ YOUR THOUGHTS CAN CHANGE YOUR LIFE *Dr. Donald Curtis*	7.00

The books listed above can be obtained from your book dealer or directly from Melvin Powers. When ordering, please remit $1.50 postage for the first book and 50¢ for each additional book.

Melvin Powers
12015 Sherman Road, No. Hollywood, California 91605